Copyright © 2016

Written by LockMarie

Edited and proofread by: LockMarie

Cover Photography by: Que's Pics

Professional photography

ISBN-13:978-1519714602

ISBN-10:1519714602

# How LockMarie Lost 65 lbs in less than 3 months

From Nov. 2010 to Feb. 2011 to this present day

I have kept the weight off!

A GIFT PRESENTED TO:

_____

FROM:

_____

DATE:

_____

# THE LOCKMARIE COLLECTION OF BOOKS INCLUDES:

1. The Tip book
2. The Poem book of poetic passion when a man loves a woman
3. Poems of passion for when a woman loves a man
4. Erotic passion for the grown and sexy (2 poem books in 1)
5. How to recognize a real friend (for ages 10 and up)?
6. Are you a deadbeat mom? Vol.1
7. The inner cries of a man- book 1 (poem book)
8. The inner cries of a man- book 2 (poem book)
9. Little King David- book 1 (children's book-my first reader)
10. I Taste Grape! (children's book)
11. Are you a deadbeat mom? Vol 2
12. How to stop dating the wrong Mr. & Ms. Right and attract the right heart and keep it!
13. A Simple beauty guide with tips for the everyday women/girls- age 9 to 99
14. I AM not who you say I am- but- I am who I say I am

COMING SOON

1. Are you a Deadbeat mom – vol. 3
2. Are you a Deadbeat mom- vol. 4
3. Are you a Deadbeat mom- vol. 5
4. The Man-U-Script- straight from the mouth of men-interviews of what men want.
5. Monster and the little boy
   (a children's book)

And many more to come

# Table of content

# Dedications

First I want to thank my Lord and Savior Jesus Christ.  If it had not been for him on my side, I do not know where or what I would be today. One thing I do know is I would not be the woman, writer, nor author I am today. Thank you for answering my prayers and giving me a 2nd chance at life.

## Ruben Benitez

PAPE' as I call you ☺ Now I had no clue what to expect when I started going to the gym.  I can just remember telling the girl at the counter, I wanted a trainer who was "about their business" and not playing around.  When she told, me you were my trainer I said, "alright I will see how long he last". Ha.

Well, all I can say is that I truly had moments when I loved to hate you- ha. You were the best trainer ever. I am so grateful for the time, dedication and drive you put forth in our sessions.  I know there is no way I could have done it without your assistance.  It was hard and sometimes I wanted to give up but you would not allow me to.  THANK YOU- THANK YOU, I will always remember you and appreciate you and all your wisdom and tips that you gave me.  You were a great motivator and encourager and you helped me push pass the pain and my limitations. I know now I can do anything I set my mind to.  To go from 200 lbs. to less than 150 lbs.

I just wanted to publicly thank you for doing your job and doing it well, you give people like me another chance to enjoy life and enjoy the bodies we are in.

## OTHER TRAINERS/COACHES

Once I lost the weight I have kept it off for the past 6 years by having a couple of phenomenal trainers/friends in my life to assist and I would like to thank them now.

# Thanks to:

**Coach Freeman**- we have known each other since elementary school and I did not even know you were a trainer.  It was great working with you and I am grateful for the exercise strategies you taught me, you were a no-nonsense coach and that is what people need to make it happen.

**Miss fit Bennett**- an amazing trainer and body builder -thanks for all your assistance and tough love -ha. You are an amazing, hardworking, determined woman and I wish you much more continued success in life. I still use the daily nutrition list you gave me and I will continue to use it.  Healthy eating and good food are a great combination; my GG would be proud of me. ☺

**Ellie N. Anthony-Perico-** A super coach, a woman that wears many hats and wears them well.  I am so blessed to have met you (even if only by social media) the tips, help and encouragement you give is priceless You have shown me it is not as hard as I thought to do what I love to do and become an expert at it. Thank you so much for just being you.  I wish you much continued success and joy in life.

# SPECIAL DEDICATIONS

**My GG,** she was my number one cheerleader, she made sure I could get to the gym and have time to work out and always helped me eat healthy and light.

She was the best example I ever had.   Her memory will forever be with me and she will always be an inspiration for me to keep moving forward and being my best. Rest in heavenly peace GG, we miss you always.....

**Que,** sweetie, you are such an amazing man and I am forever grateful to have you on my team.  You push me forward and assist me in reaching all my goals and I love you for that. When I don't think, I can do it, you keep reminding me I can. You even change your eating habits to compliment mine and I know sometimes you might not feel like doing things but you are so selfless and make sure I am staying on track and on point.   You have shown me what true love is. Thank you, baby, and because of you I will forever perfect this body of mine to make you smile and feel proud to have me on your arm. Love, you always...

**David,** my heart, my reason I work so hard and do as much as I do to be a good example. Son mama is so proud of you and how you are growing into a great young man.  You love people and it shows.  You are kind and gentle and have a loving spirit.  My big gentle giant you are. I love to see you exercise and always ask to eat healthy foods. It makes me feel good that you are watching and learning and want to be a healthy and fit young man. Never give up, never quit. You can and will reach all your goals in life and continue to make me proud. I love you and cannot wait to see the man you will grow to be.

# Introduction

I am just an everyday woman here to show other every day women that it is possible and it can be done. I am so tired of us using the excuse I cannot afford to, I am not a celebrity, I just do not have the time. No excuses ladies, the excuses stop here.

Well, it all started back in 2006 when I started gaining weight. I went from 98lbs to 115, 120, 130lbs and it felt like I was still growing. I got pregnant with my son and went to 160 and after giving birth I kept growing ha. I ended up a whopping 200 or more lbs. in less than 2 years, UGH! I could not stand looking at myself in the mirror. It was horrific. The doctor warned me it was NOT the baby, it was me. I promised myself that I was not going to be one of those ladies going through life blaming the weight on baby fat (and the kid is 29 years old ha). I had to make a change, I was not feeling good about it at all. I did not fit in my clothing, nor did they look cute nor did I like how I looked in clothing and I do not even want to mention how I looked naked ugh.

I was not comfortable being large, I had been a small framed girl my entire life, so this was shocking and mind blowing for me. It may be cool for some people, but it was NOT cool for me. I had to make a change. So, that is who I want to speak to in this book. Those women who do not like it and want change.

Along with a big life transition that was another major MUST in my life, I decided that the best revenge was to be better, look better and do better than I did before.

So, I joined a gym, I got a trainer and made it happen. It was not easy. I will not lie and say it was, nope it was hard work and took complete determination and commitment. I had not worked out in over 6 years so it took a lot for me to do it, but I was committed and determined to snap back and get back control of my life.

## Beginning Steps

Sometimes in life, we allow others to distract us and get us off track, but when that happens we cannot blame anyone but ourselves. I was tired of playing the blame game so I took back my control, and every day I now look back and thank God that I did. It was one of the best decisions I ever made in my life.

I pray this book assist and helps hundreds even millions of you to better your life and find your better self. You can be at your best and love yourself and love what you see daily. If you want to be healthy, fit and on point, you can do it, never let anyone make you feel you are too big or too out of shape, there is no such thing. It does not exist. Those are just lame excuses; you have the power within you to make it happen and make a change. YOU CAN DO IT-- I DID IT -AND SO CAN YOU!!!!!! Here are some beginning steps for you to remember that aided me in my successful life change:

**Prayer**: In everything you do, always include God and he will always give you what you need to do, and how to complete your task. What works for one person might not work for you, but prayer always works for those that apply it. I believe God is the creator of us all, so if he made us, he knows the very things you need to do, to be your best, but you must first ask him. I always pray, I have been doing so since I was a child. The older I get the more I do it. I told God I was tired of being big and having my thighs rub together and sweating and being musty ugh, some things are just NOT cute, I don't care what nobody says. The bible tells us "In everything that you do- talk to God about it and he will direct you in the way you should go"– (Proverbs 3 verse 6- LockMarie translation)

**A made-up mind**: Anything you go to do in life, you must make up your mind to do it. When the alarm clock goes off in the morning, if you do not make up your mind to get out the bed, guess what, you will lay there. I know I have done it many times before. You must focus on it and keep your mind on whatever the task is at hand. It starts in the mind. It is always a thought first. If you do not think about it, 9 times out of 10 you will never do it. I know there have been times when I wanted to eat healthy, but my mind was not made up and as I ate the donuts and cookies, I was thinking "I should not be eating all these sweets". A lot of times because it tastes so good, or feels so good, it makes you focus more on the feeling than on what you know in your mind is the right thing to do.

**Determination:** You must be focused and determined to do it. It is very easily said, but not easily done. It will be difficult at times but it will be worth it, believe me. Do not give up, stay in there and hold on until the end. It is like being in a race and you are running and you know that if you finish the race you will receive a medal. Whether it is a 1st place or a 50th place, you have something to look forward to. That is the way you should stay determined when it comes to your health and getting to the weight that is your target. The bible also says "Be ye steadfast, and unmovable", determined- (I Corinthians 15 verse 58-LockMarie translation)

**Hard work:** No matter what in life you try to accomplish, it will take work. Most things in life we desire and want, do not come easy. Get ready to work and work hard. I will never lie and say it was easy for me to lose the weight. I got tired, I got mad, I got frustrated. That is what happens when you are on a job at times, it gets hard. If it was easy, everyone would do it. Hard work is not for everyone. I know some people that only like things easy. They never want to work hard for anything. They want everything handed to them the easy way. Well those people need not apply here.

**Dedication: DO NOT GIVE UP.** Be steadfast and unmovable. It will take time, it will not happen overnight, but if you keep on keeping on, it SHALL come to pass.

This takes me back to my favorite book, the bible- I Corinthians 15 verse 58 "Be steadfast, unmovable, always abounding in work, for your labor is not in vain in the lord". Do not stop until your goal has been reached. I can remember when I got my job, I was dedicated. I wanted to make a year. I had never been on a real job and I was determined to be dedicated and make my year. Well now 20 years later, I see how being dedicated works. I know some people who have had many jobs and lost them all. I know many people who have had many relationships and have not been dedicated. You must be dedicated to everything in life in order to complete anything. Do not give up.

**Consistency-Daily:** Do it daily, hourly and on schedule. You must have a schedule. Use this book and journal your progress and your daily journey. Take it one day at a time. Start small with baby steps, but be consistent with whatever you do. Start off 1 day a week and be consistent. For a month, do 1 day a week, then the next month, add another day a week. Keep going and adding each week and the more constant you are, the more you will accomplish.

**Motivation:** Sometimes if you do not have someone else to motivate you, you must motivate yourself. I did not have many cheerleaders on my journey, so I kept my mind focused on my goal and I made it. Trainers are great motivators, but if you cannot afford a trainer, go online and google other success stories of people that have done what you are trying to do and let them motivate you. Follow those in the fitness world online and look at their pictures to get a mental picture of what you would like to accomplish. Make it realistic and stay motivated.

**Will power:** You must have the inner drive to do it because sometimes that is all you must push you through it. Never give up and give in, even if you cheat or stop, you can always start again. Each day is another day to get back on track. Like the little engine says, "I think I can, I think I can". Yes, you can, if you have the will power, you can do it. One thing you must do is shut off other people and negative influences that come to distract you. Stay focused and hold on. How bad do you want it? You are the main determination here.

**Structure:** Map out your routine, your daily schedule and menus. Always have written down what you are going to do for the day and what you wish to achieve. Never leave it up in the air. Always follow a schedule. This is a good way to stay on track. Some people can do this without thinking, but most people need to write things down. I know many people who need structure in their lives. They are so care free and have no schedule and no sense of time or structure. They are late to everything and do not know how to be responsible. Then they get mad and frustrated when things in life never turn out the way they want. They do not plan, so it cannot turn out the way they planned, when they have no plan.

I have had this happen to me too at various times in life. I know there were times when I should have been more structured and I was not. I had to make up my mind and structure my time and then everything else fell into place.

# DAILY JOURNAL

# Normal withdrawals

You will go through changes, your body will feel funny and weird, and you may even have mood swings ha. All of this is normal, and it varies from person to person. I know I had a big withdrawal when I stopped eating sugar. Woo, my body was like- hold up and wait a minute! I was also a big chocolate fan and when I stopped for about a month, I thought "wow this must be what an addict feels like when they do not have their drug for a while".  You must remember you are not a super hero and your body is not a cartoon.

Remember the following:

**BE HUMAN:** You are not a super hero, you are human. Do not over do or push yourself too hard. Baby steps are best. Like I stated earlier, if you cheat or stop for a while or even get discouraged, that is okay, just do not give up.  Take a break, re-group and then get back to it.

**MAKE IT FUN:** I say this because anything that is too much like work, will not be fun or something you will want to do, or even enjoy doing.  So make a game out of it.  Get a visual of what you want to look like and please make it realistic.

**ENCOURAGE YOURSELF:** Give yourself daily compliments and pep talks. Sometimes other people may see your progress but they will not admit it or compliment you- so encourage yourself. Look in the mirror and say "girl you looking good, I am so proud of you."

Just because others do not acknowledge it does NOT mean it is not happening or visible. A lot of people just do not know how to compliment or encourage others. Let's just be honest here- a lot of people just do not want to ha. They see you looking good but as I have come to recognize, it is easier for some to hate or be jealous- which I say is what other women do when they have not been taught to compliment others.  They do not know how to say- I like that or you look nice, so they hate.   It takes too much work and effort to smile and be nice so they take the easy way out. Remember some people do not like hard work.

These are just a few of the many things I used to make it from the start of my journey to the end.

I wrote this book to help others realize that it is possible to lose weight and it does not take a long period BUT it will take self-denial and consistency.

One important note that we all need to realize is that, everyone is different.  Each person's body responds differently.

Along with the tips and secrets I give you, you also may have to find things that will only work for you.

Have you ever seen those that go on diets, work out and still never lose weight? It is because they must find out what works for their body along with the regular normal remedies.

One thing that is important is to do your research.  Find a professional nutritionist that can give you the foods to eat and what to cut back on.  Contrary to popular belief, you do not always have to stop eating foods for good. If you are an everyday person and you are just working a regular job and just trying to lose a few pounds or tone up, you might just need to monitor yourself and watch your calorie intake.

All my life I was a small framed person, it did not matter what I ate or how I ate, because my metabolism was so fast it was ridiculous. I wore 98 pounds for about 16 years of my life.

Then I had my son in 2008 and the doctor warned me while I was pregnant that my baby was not that big so most of the weight I was carrying was that, weight. They told me the foods to stay away from which included most if not all my favorites. Such as cheese, milk, mayonnaise and fast foods. Well, I was a fast food Queen and always loved to add cheese and mayo to my foods. So, I heard the doctor and made up my mind I was not going to listen- ha.

Well I paid for it. I ended up 200 pounds or more.  Now for most of you, you may not see anything wrong with that, but you must remember I was always small.  I was not use to carrying around weight, I was devastated and in complete shock.

I went from sizes 0, 2, 4, petite-small, x-small and smalls to get this-, sizes ranging from 16 to 18 and 2XL, 3XL. I did not like who I had turned into. I would look in the mirror and think, who are you, and what have you done to my body.  The person I was with at that time was not any help either. They over cooked, over ate and never encouraged me to lose any weight.  Side note ladies, it is not always because a man loves you that he will accept you as is, he does not want you to better yourself sometimes and wants to keep you down. Let's NOT get it twisted. Real love does accept you as you are, BUT if you can stand to better yourself they will tell you in love (as my now current fiancé does often and I love him more for that)

It was not until I was tired of being sick and tired that I made a change, in more ways than one.

Finally, I had made up my mind (because that is where it starts) to make a major change in my life. I tease and when women ask me what I did to lose the weight, I always say, the first thing I did was I lost like over 200 some pounds of a man, (sometimes ladies that is the 1$^{st}$ step) change your environment and your surroundings and your life is guaranteed to get better.

I knew it was time for a great transition. I got on my knees and prayed and I told God I was tired and I was ready for a change.

I made up my mind and was focused on getting a better life and a better body for myself.  A lot of times when you are stressed, depressed, upset, angry, controlled and disappointed in your relationships, it will have a great impact on your appearance and your health. You will never be at your best physically if you are messed up mentally and emotionally. (my opinion of course) In November of 2010 I enrolled in a gym and got a personal trainer.  I had like 6 weeks of training and sessions.  I went almost 4 times a week and changed a lot of my eating habit. Another major point was -I did NOT eat after 7 pm nor did I eat large portions anymore.

# TIPS TO CHANGE YOUR BODY WEIGHT/SHAPE

## Watch your portions:

## Portions control -portion control-portion control!

If you always eat 3 pieces of chicken, cut it down to 1.
If you always eat 4 slices of pizza, only eat 2.
If you always eat a large bowl of cereal, use a small or mini bowl.
Whatever amount of food you usually eat, cut it down in half. This is a great start to a greater body.  You do not have to go cold turkey unless you can handle it. Do not make it a task or work, make it a gift.  You want to enjoy it, for it to be successful.

## Cut down or cut out certain foods:

Along with the portions, you should also cut down greatly or even cut out sugar and caffeine intake completely.  I stopped drinking sodas for almost 4 years.  That acid/sugar in those sodas go straight to the belly, not to mention it messes up many normal functions of the body.  Google sodas and see the world out there.  I still cannot believe as a child I use to drink them like water, ugh. Thank God I grew up and learned so I could break that normal bad habit. My son has NEVER had a soda in my presence or on my watch. He is 7 years old now and if I am there he will not. I want him to start out right to stay right.

Now I am a sugar and chocolate junky. I love chocolate, so what I had to do was to monitor myself and when I would eat at least 4 to 5 snickers and 2 to 3 packs of donuts and cookies a week, I had to cut it down to maybe 1 snicker and 1 pack of sweets a week.  There was no way I was completely giving it up- haa.  I just need to keep it real and honest.

Dairy is another group that you should avoid (but if you are like me that is not an option ha) so cut down as much as possible.

Now there have been times where I would go cold turkey for about 6 months to a year at a time because I had a certain weight goal or shape goal in mind. I have worked with some of the best trainers and nutritionist out there (in my opinion) so that now I know what to do, to get what results.

I am grateful for this knowledge because it keeps me satisfied with my body and my results. Even though most people are mainly concerned with weight lost, it is health- that is to be your number one goal.

Good health is very important. Once you eat healthy, the weight will and can be maintained.

I saw a lot of my family members have strokes and heart attacks and even die from poor health. I was determined to live a long healthy full life so I made a change. I have a variety of foods to eat to maintain good health and a consistent weight. No one likes to fluctuate from one weight to another. We all want to remain one size or another. Well to do so. You must eat a certain way.

You should always consult a doctor before trying any new meal plans or diets. I am only giving suggestions that helped and aided me in my transition.

**Special tips:** there are a couple of other things that have added in my health and fitness. They serve a lot of great purposes, please do your research and see how and if it can assist you also. We all are different so you must see what works for you.

- Apple Cider vinegar- I love using a certain brand (I will not mention since I am not getting paid to do so ha) but I pour some of this in various drinks I use daily. Google, it and you will see the great purpose it has on your life and your body.
- Coconut Oil- a new found love of mine, that not only helps my health but my skin and hair.
- Olive oil- I have always been in love with this cause I am a church girl so it serves many uses ha..
- Water and lemon-why didn't somebody tell my mama about lemon in water as a kid ha. I have been drinking water all my life, but that would have made it even tastier.

## Breakfast

I was a full breakfast eater for years. I mean, pancakes, eggs, bacon, hash browns.  French toast, bacon, grits, biscuits, syrup.  I loved breakfast.

So, it was a little difficult changing my habits, but I knew I wanted to live long and healthy so I did.

Now I always have a day when I enjoy my favorites at least once a month or so, but I have learned to enjoy new favorites.

-oatmeal- small portion with a little honey

-boiled egg whites only

-bananas and other fruits

-small portion of grits

-certain breakfast bars

-certain breakfast drinks

-if I have a bagel, I only eat one side

-lean turkey patties/turkey bacon

-green smoothies or drinks with veggies/fruits


## LIST ANY OTHER BREAKFAST FOODS YOU MAY WANT TO USE.

_____

_____

_____

_____

_____

_____

_____

_____

_____

_____

_____

_____

_____

## Lunch

Now this was the hard part for me, since I work 8 hours a day, lunch is a very anticipated meal for me. I can skip breakfast or even a dinner but I must have my lunch.

So instead of my regular hot dogs, hamburgers, pizzas, and sandwiches. I began eating salads. I know you are frowning, but salads are a great meal for lunch.

It is not too heavy and not too light. You can add turkey meats or chicken or even tuna.

Now I am not saying I did not eat fast food, but I cut down a lot. As of now, I probably only eat out maybe once a month, when I go out with a coworker. What I normally do now, is I make my lunch like a good girl ha. I work in an office which means I sit most of the day, so the "office spread" is very much alive. When you have a sit-down desk job you need to watch your food intake.

I also make sure I have little health snacks and every 2 hours I have one. A fruit, nuts, or health bar and then after lunch I have something to hold me over until I get home for dinner.

Lunch foods I enjoy:

-salads with chicken or turkey chunks
-half of sandwich
-soup
-fruit
-protein drinks/smoothies (low sugar, even better no sugar)
-extra lean turkey meat/patties
-jasmine brown/white rice/brown rice
-skinless chicken breast
List other healthy/low fat foods you think you could enjoy at lunch:

_____
_____
_____
_____
_____
_____
_____
_____
_____
_____
_____
_____
_____
_____
_____
_____
_____
_____
_____
_____
_____

## DINNER

Now it is very important that you do not eat late. I say do not eat after 7 pm but I will give you 7:30 pm. Try your hardest, not to eat too close to bed time, if you do make sure it is something light. The only time it is good to eat after this time, is when you are on an every 2.5 to 2-hour program and gallon of water intake. Sometimes you must jumpstart your metabolism again.

I do not eat a lot of red meat.
I usually eat fish, turkey or chicken.
I even cut down on my ground beef intake.
Turkey patties and turkey meats are great substitutes for those foods.
No steak, no fried chicken (I cannot remember the last time I had fried chicken) or please limit as much as possible.
I like pasta and spaghetti so I will have a small portion maybe once a month.
I love veggies, so I eat mainly all green veggies like peas, broccoli, spinach and green salads. You must still be careful with some veggies, due to sugar intake.
I cut out the canned veggies all together.

More dinner foods I enjoy:

-turkey parts
-soups
-salads
-baked chicken
-grilled chicken
-jasmine rice/brown rice
-baked potatoes (with nothing added but a little butter)
-pasta with little to no sauce
-asparagus
-green veggies
-fish- tilapia or sometimes patties
Google is your friend so check on line for more good eats.

_____
_____
_____
_____
_____
_____
_____
_____
_____
_____
_____
_____
_____
_____
_____
_____

## Now Desserts –

This is where I get in trouble.
I love sweets as I stated earlier.
It is hard sometimes but I do make it ever so often- ha.
There are always things you can snack on like:
-jello
-popcorn
-fruit
-pudding
-fat free popsicles


Now if you have the munchies and the "I got to have it" as I do sometimes, it is best that you watch your portion intake.
Small portions are always best if you cannot go cold turkey.
Believe it or not, you do not have to have a dessert. You can just go with dinner; I know we have this notion that we must have dessert but you do not have to. ☺
I also have my success story of my weight lost on a site called shapefit.com. it is a great place to go and see and read other people success stories and get tips and information that could help you in your journey to a healthier body.
Now you may still feel like you cannot do it. I want you to know that you can do this. It is not as hard as it seems.
If you have a mental picture of what you want to look like, and make sure it is realistic. Start small, when I lost all the weight I lost I was not aiming for any weight, I just wanted to lose weight.  The weight did not come off first, but inches did.  I began to lose inches around my waist first.  The scale said the same thing because the fat was shifting into muscle and moving into other parts of the body.  I was becoming proportioned.
No matter what, stick to it and do not give up or become discouraged.
You can do this. I believe in you.

# Exercise/fitness

Now this is where many people mess up. In my opinion because this book is only that, my opinion, a lot of people are exercising when all they need to do is change the way they eat.

Most people do not see any results because they eat all kinds of foods and amount of foods at all hours of the day and then go to the gym as if that is going to do something.

Sorry you are wasting your time. Exercise is used to tone up fat and the muscles after you have lost the weight. For those that do not have weight, they go to the gym for the muscles to stay in place.

I see so many people at the gym and I sort of feel sorry because the gyms are taking their money and not explaining to them it is just that, a waste of money. You would be better off walking, or doing the stairs in your neighborhood.

Simple is best, but I would recommend everyone pay for a trainer at least once in your life time.  The knowledge they give you will be priceless and last you a lifetime.  Ask all the questions you can and get all the information out of them you can and then once the sessions are up, you can use that knowledge and stay on the right path in life from then out.

Another thing I notice is a lot of women, especially, they lose weight but they never firm it up.

If you are going to lose weight, then tone it up. Why lose it so it can just hang and shift to other areas and you are still carrying it around.  Go to a gym, or walk and do some sort of exercises to firm that flab up.  It is just waving and flapping and you look like you are in between stages. I know, I was there, and I did not like to have my arm waving and I was already done. I did not like my belly jiggling and my legs rubbing together.  In my opinion, some things are just not cute nor sexy. Extra skin and weight lost should not stick around but it should be toned up and tightened, so that all your hard work can be seen at its best.

(while writing this) I had just come back from a trip visiting my dad in Oklahoma City and I was so proud of him, he is 39 now (61) ha, and he goes to the gym at least 4 times a week and does 40 minutes to an hour on the treadmill. He has stopped eating bread and a lot of things that most people cannot give up.  He looks great and is an inspiration to others in his community.

He would always laugh at people and talk about them for going to the gym but he knows now, that as you get older, sometimes you must do things differently.

Some of you may say it is expensive to go to a gym or to hire a trainer, well I say most of the things you purchase with your money, you probably do not need. This is something that will benefit you and your family for a lifetime so it is a great investment. Save if you must, most gyms will let you make payments, do not say no before you try.

FAITH WITHOUT WORKS IS NULL AND VOID

EAT RIGHT, EXERCISE, AND THINK RIGHT ABOUT IT ALL.

You are your worst enemy.  If you want to change your life, your happiness and your future, then you must make a change.

No one else can do it for you.  IT IS ALL UP TO YOU.

Do not get mad at other women that do it and look good, you could do the same thing.  Give it a try and I guarantee you will be glad you did.

### Being over Weight is NOT healthy- in LockMarie's opinion

I know a lot of people are happy and satisfied at the size they are, and that is okay, but is it healthy. No one is saying you must be a size 2 or 4 but whatever you are, make it healthy. A lot of problems you face in life, is due to the extra weight that you should lose. If 20 pounds made the difference between your life span being 5 to 10 years longer, would you lose the weight? Sometimes you need to look at it as such. Your body was designed to function a certain way and if you are not allowing it to do so, you are making things harder on yourself.

Forget looking like others, and fitting into tight clothes, do it for your health, do it for your kids, so you can live to see them grow up and have kids. Do it so you can enjoy life and not just live day to day with regrets.

You are missing out on so much in life, just talk to anyone who was overweight and then lost it and see the difference and how they see life differently and enjoy it more. You can try and overlook and ignore it if you want, but it will catch up with you sooner or later.

So be smart and act and be healthy and live a long prosperous life in a body that you love. I know you are saying you love the body you have, you are supposed to say that, but take it from someone who been there, I guarantee you will love the new body even better.

I can remember when I was larger, I was miserable. When it was hot it was HOT, I would sweat in places that were disgusting. I was just uncomfortable and did not like the body I was in. My clothes did not fit right and I had to try on everything I bought before I bought it to make sure it fit. I am at my best when I am happy and I am happiest when I am fit and healthy. Now like I said this book is for those who know where they are now in their size and health is not where they should be, if you like where you are, then more power to you. This book will only help those that it was written to assist, those willing and ready to change for the better.

NOTES

# HEALTH ISSUES

## Not what the doctor ordered

There are many health issues related to being overweight.

I know may people personally who doctors have told to lose weight or prepare to die. Eat healthy or prepare to die. Maybe not that blunt but that is what they were told.

Heart attacks and strokes.

These are too issues that have affected my family personally. The first thing that the doctor wants to know is how is their daily diets. How is the salt intake, the sugar intake? They check their cholesterol levels and blood pressure. Do they drink water and how much water do they drink? Which brings me to my next point.

# Water is a must

The past 12 or more years I have done my best to make sure my water intake is accurate.  It keeps me flushed and it keeps me hydrated.  My skin is clear and I feel good.

There are many ways to calculate how much water you should drink personally so please do your research and make sure you take in the right amount, daily.

I rarely drink juice now; I use water more than anything. I will use crystal light packages and always put lemon slices and sometimes even cucumbers and orange slices, for flavor.

I can honestly say I probably have had 1 soda this entire year.  I truly have cut it out of my daily menu.  I will advise anyone to do so.  Sodas are not good.  Now I know that caffeine is addicting and a few years back I had went almost 2 years without one and then one day I just had to have it, so my fiancé went and got me an orange flavored soda and when it hit my throat it felt like I had took a swig of some apple cider vinegar straight haa.. it burned so and the taste was not pleasant any more.

So, you can understand my shock and devastation in gaining weight, here are some before the before shots. I was a small young girl and lady up till around age 32..

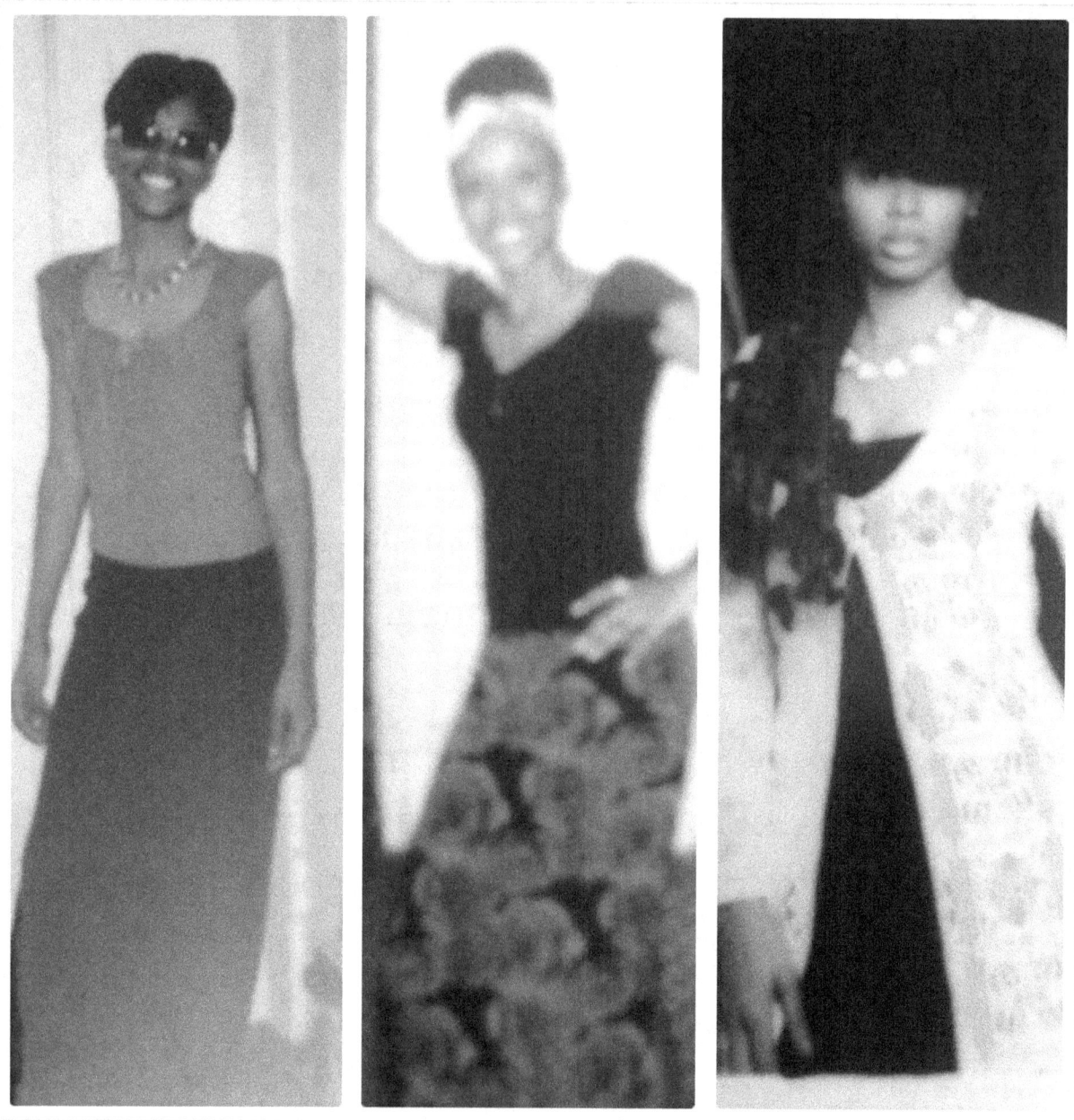

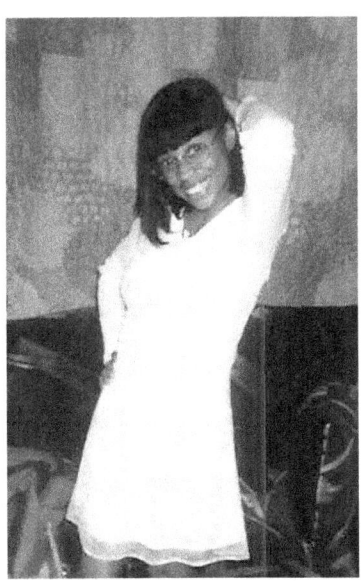

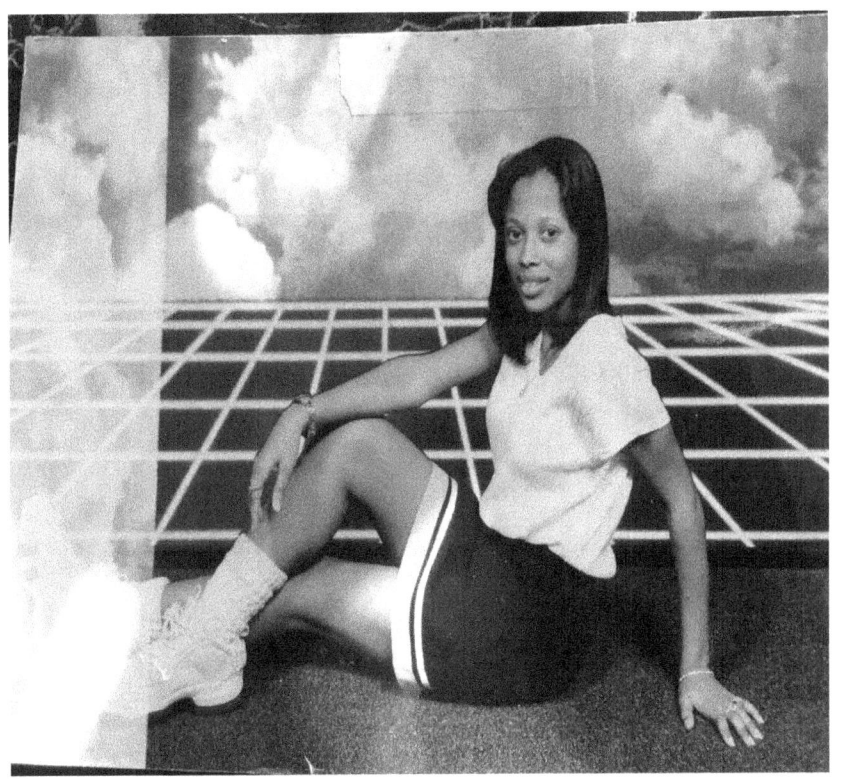

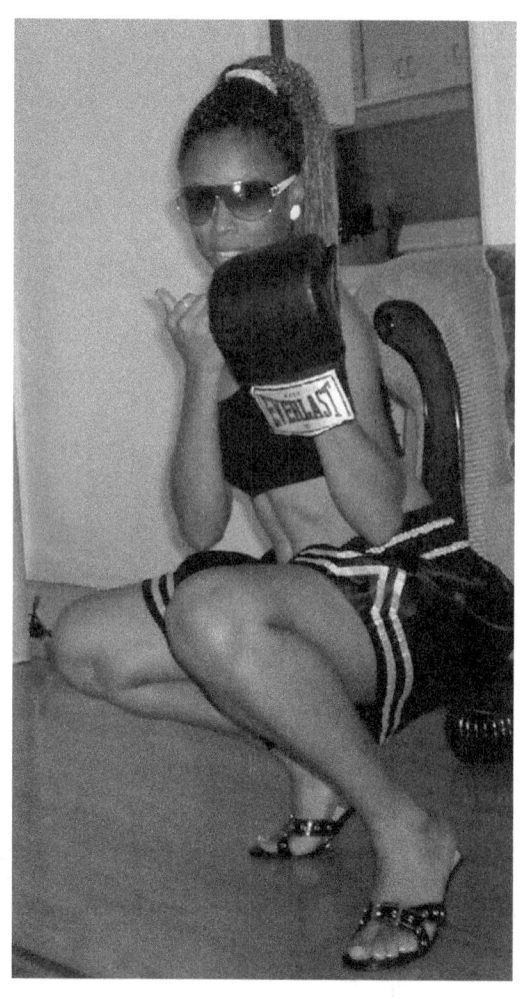

So, to go from this in 2006 to what you are about to see, you would have been in shock too ha….

# pictures-from 2009 to Nov. 2010

## At 190 almost 200 plus pounds

I did not take many full body shot pictures- since I was not comfortable being as the doctor called it "obese" for my height. It is very important to have before pictures so that when you look back you can see your progress and understand that your hard work and dedication did pay off.

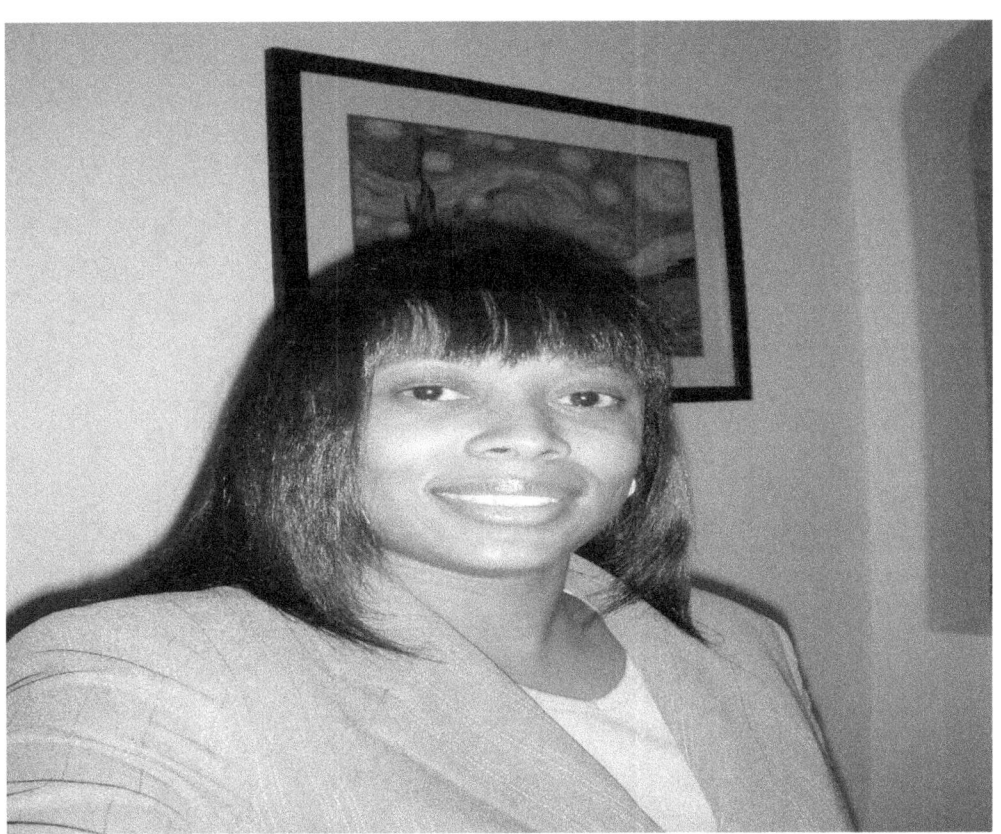

# Look at those chubby cheeks

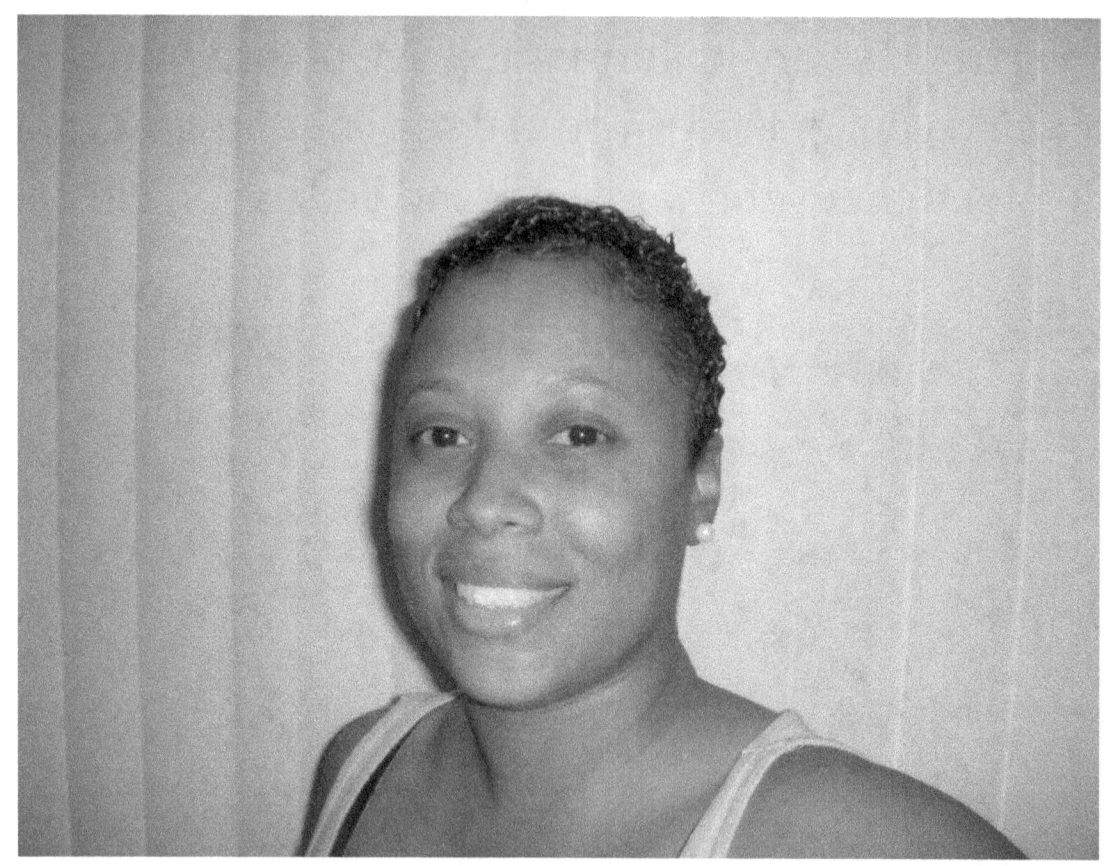

In my defense on this one I think I was pregnant ha

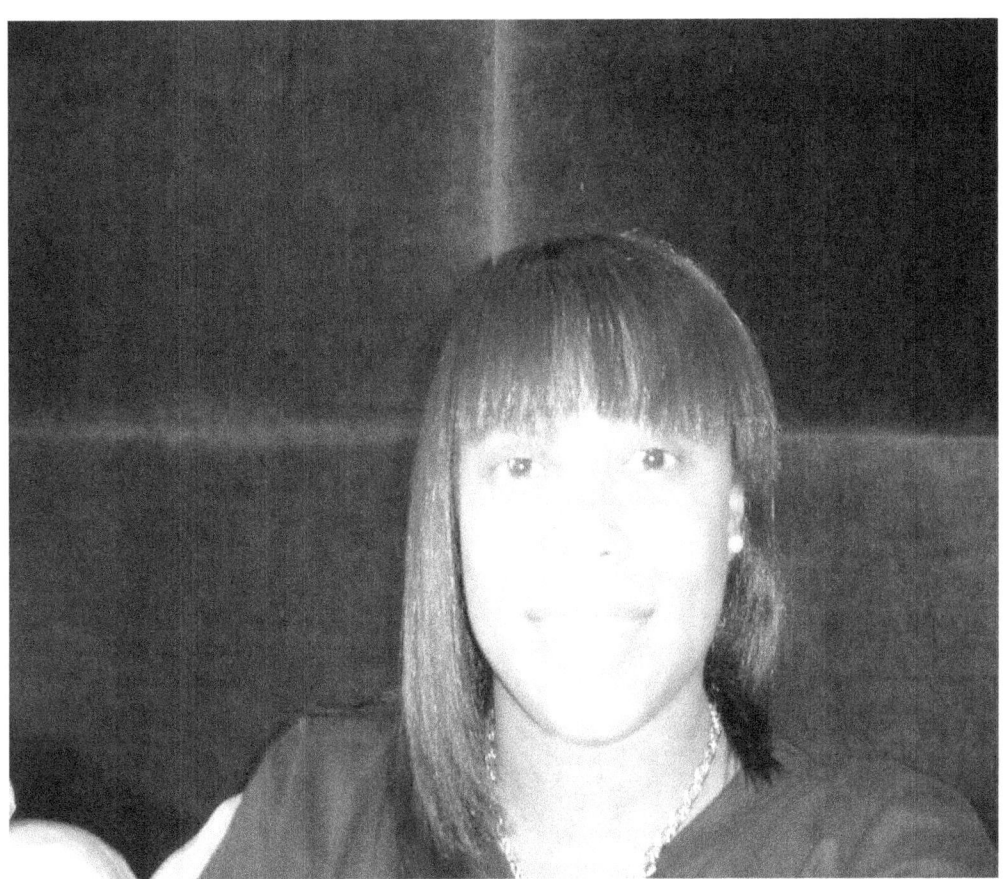

I look like a swollen balloon wow; I cannot believe that was me

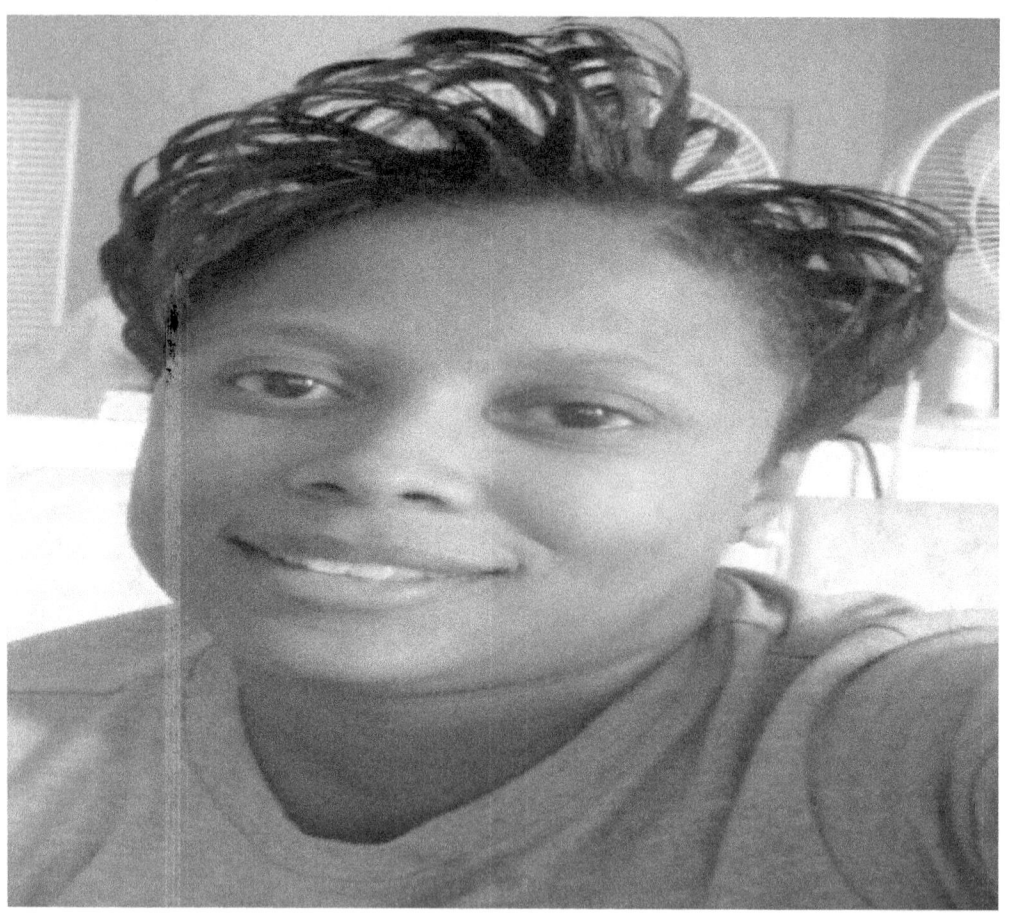

Just out of shape and big, wow.

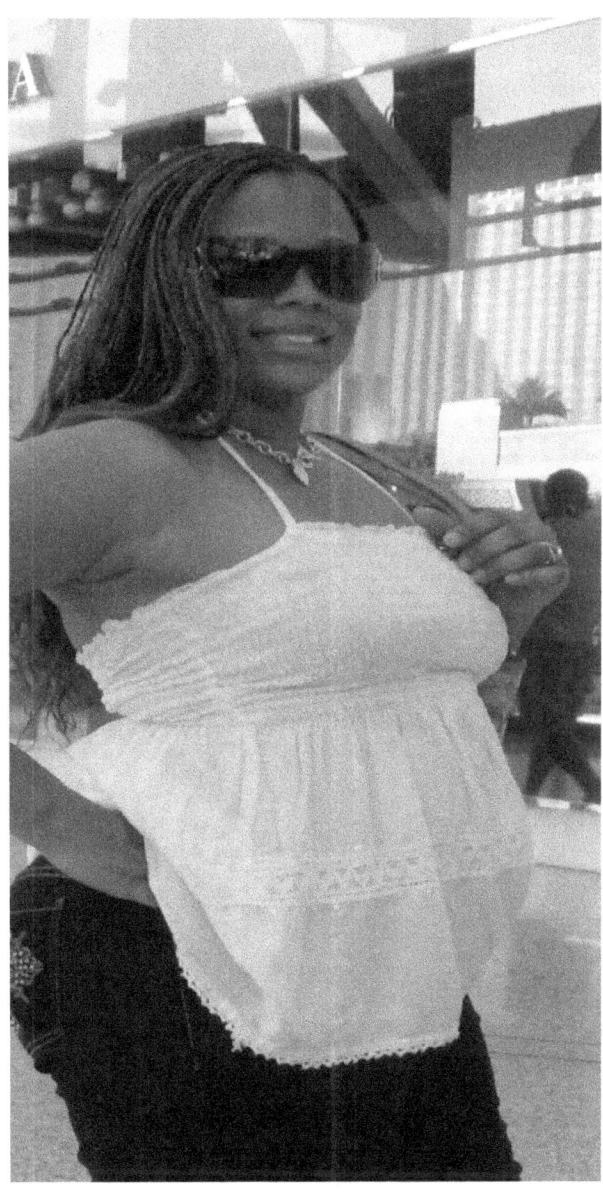

My son was at least almost 1 years old here

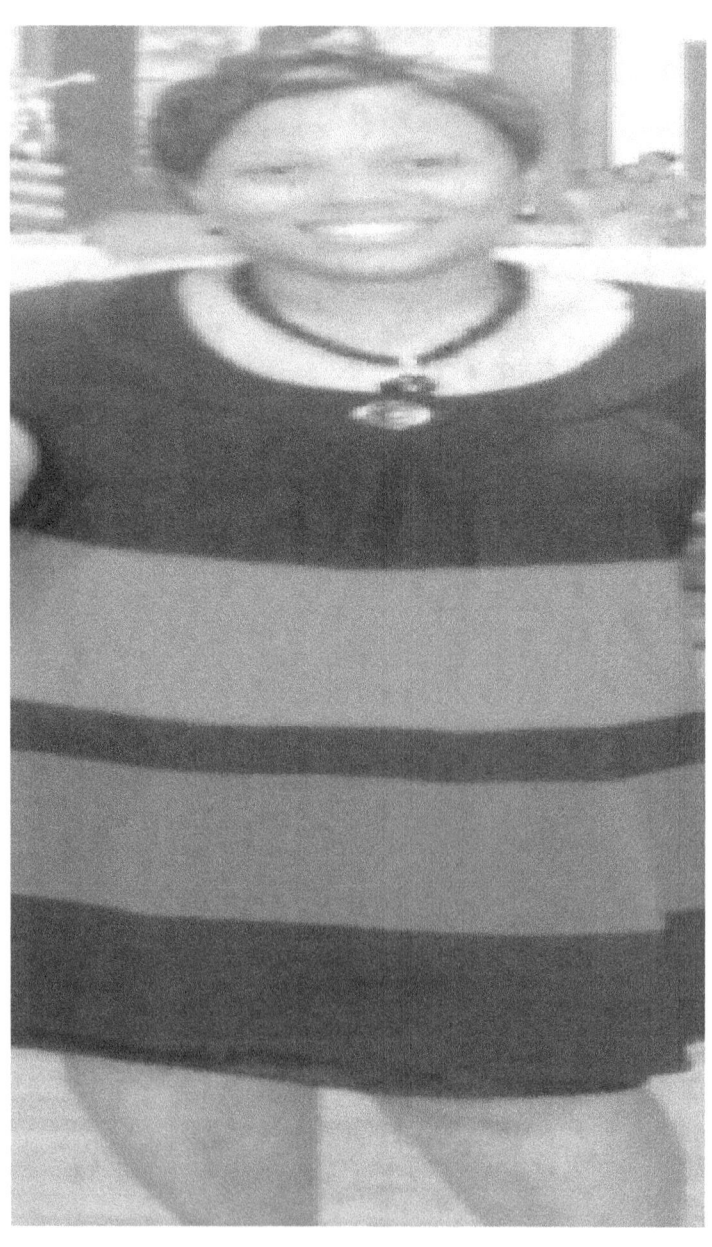

My mom and I looking like twins ☺

(I am in the light color without the pearls)

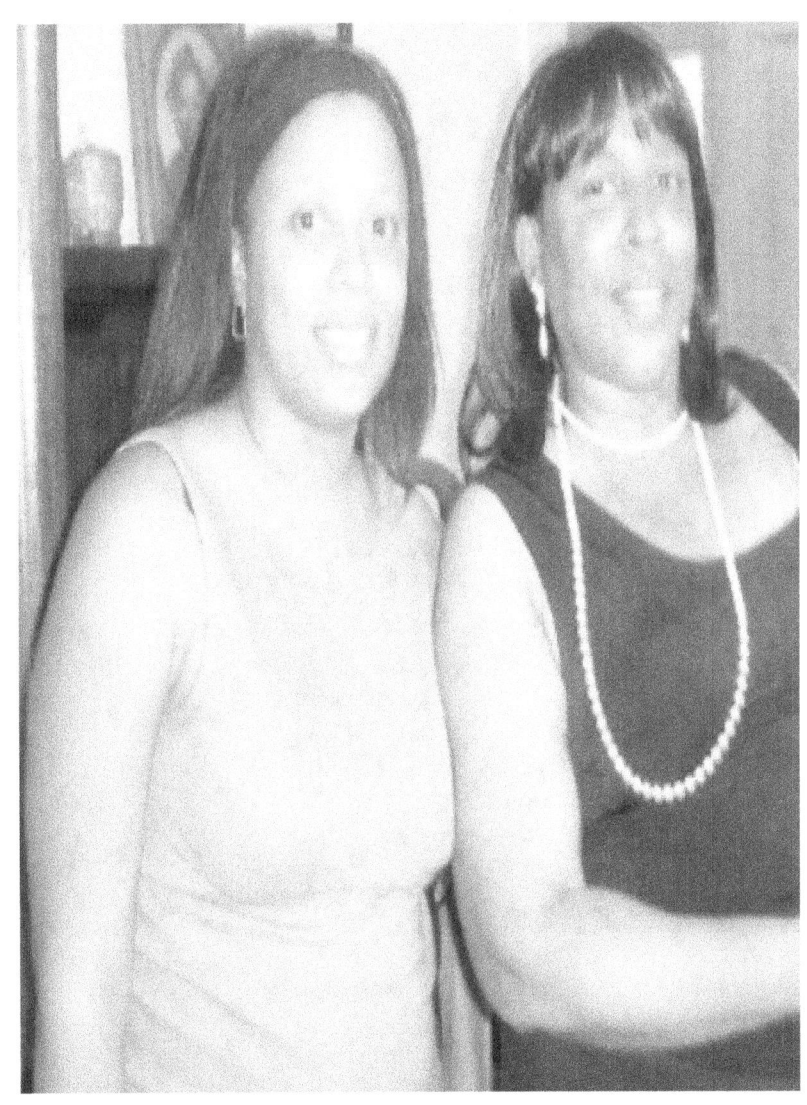

When I bought this dress, I bought it a small size to lose weight

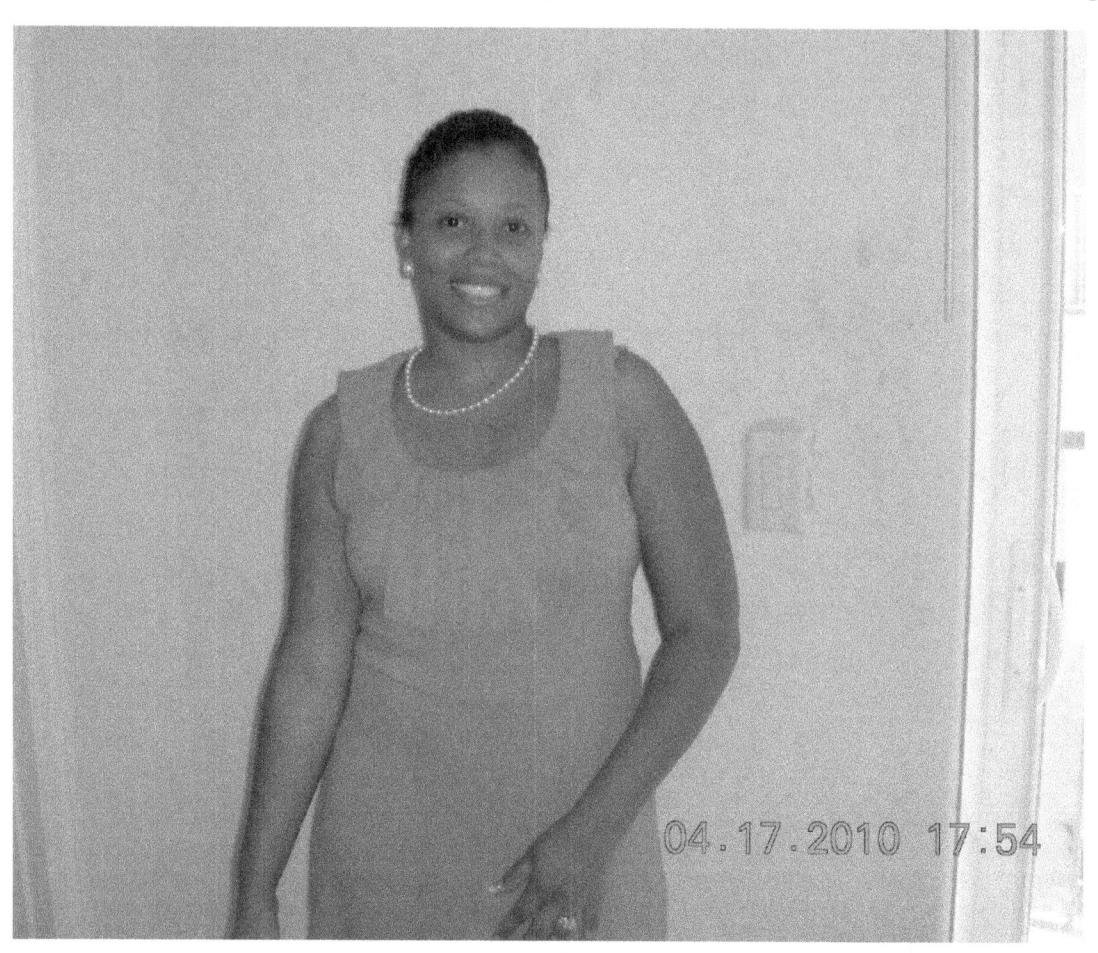

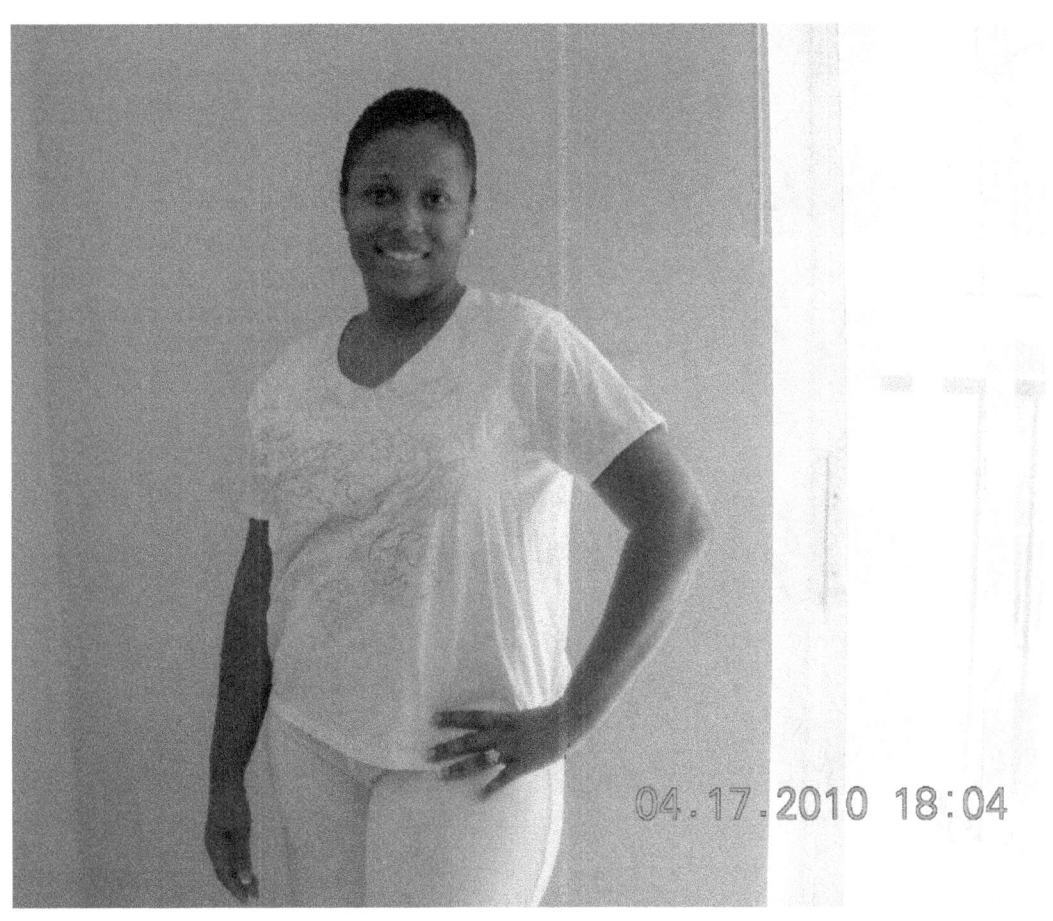

04.17.2010 18:04

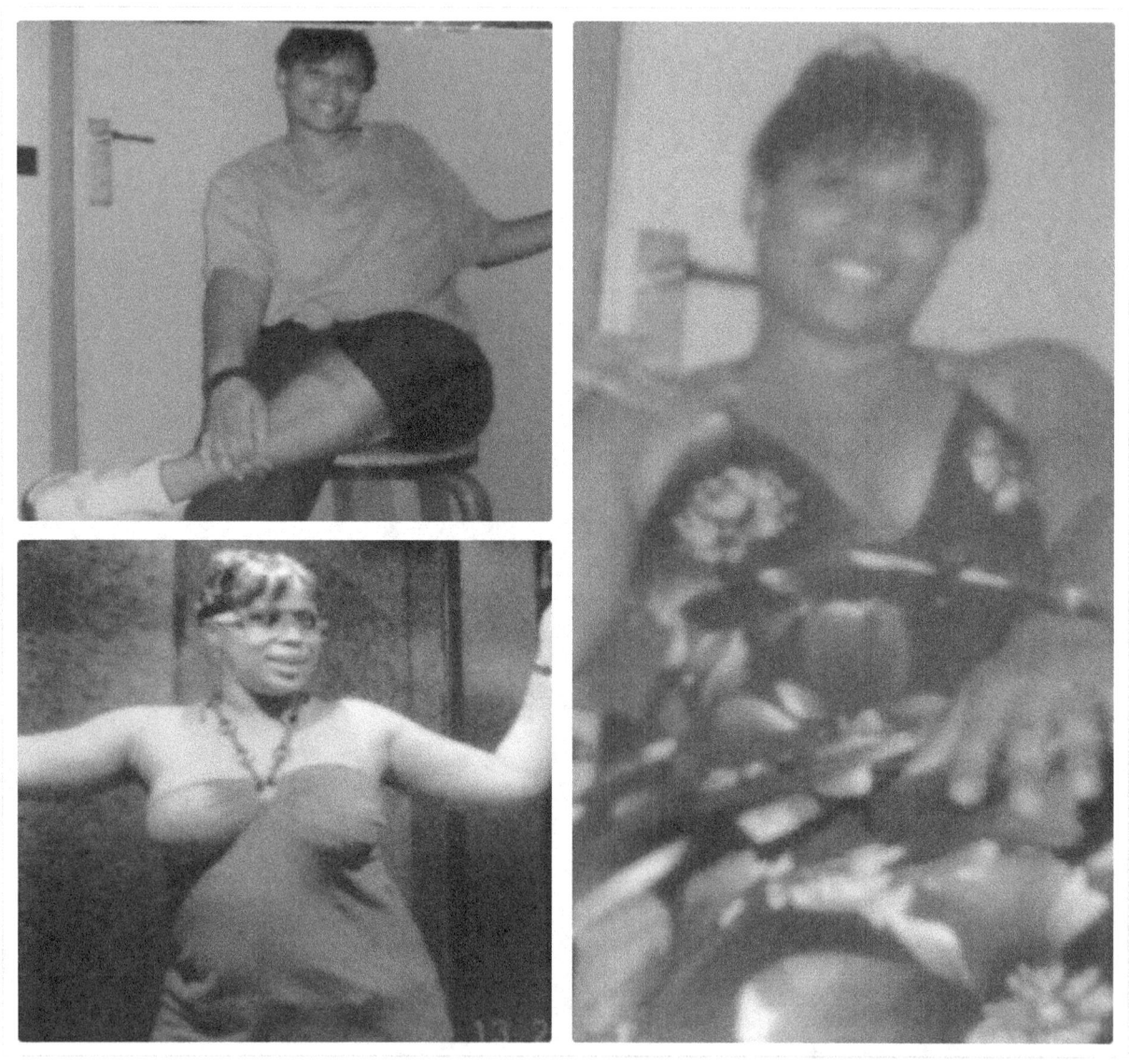

Feb. 2010-
right before I made up my mind enough was enough

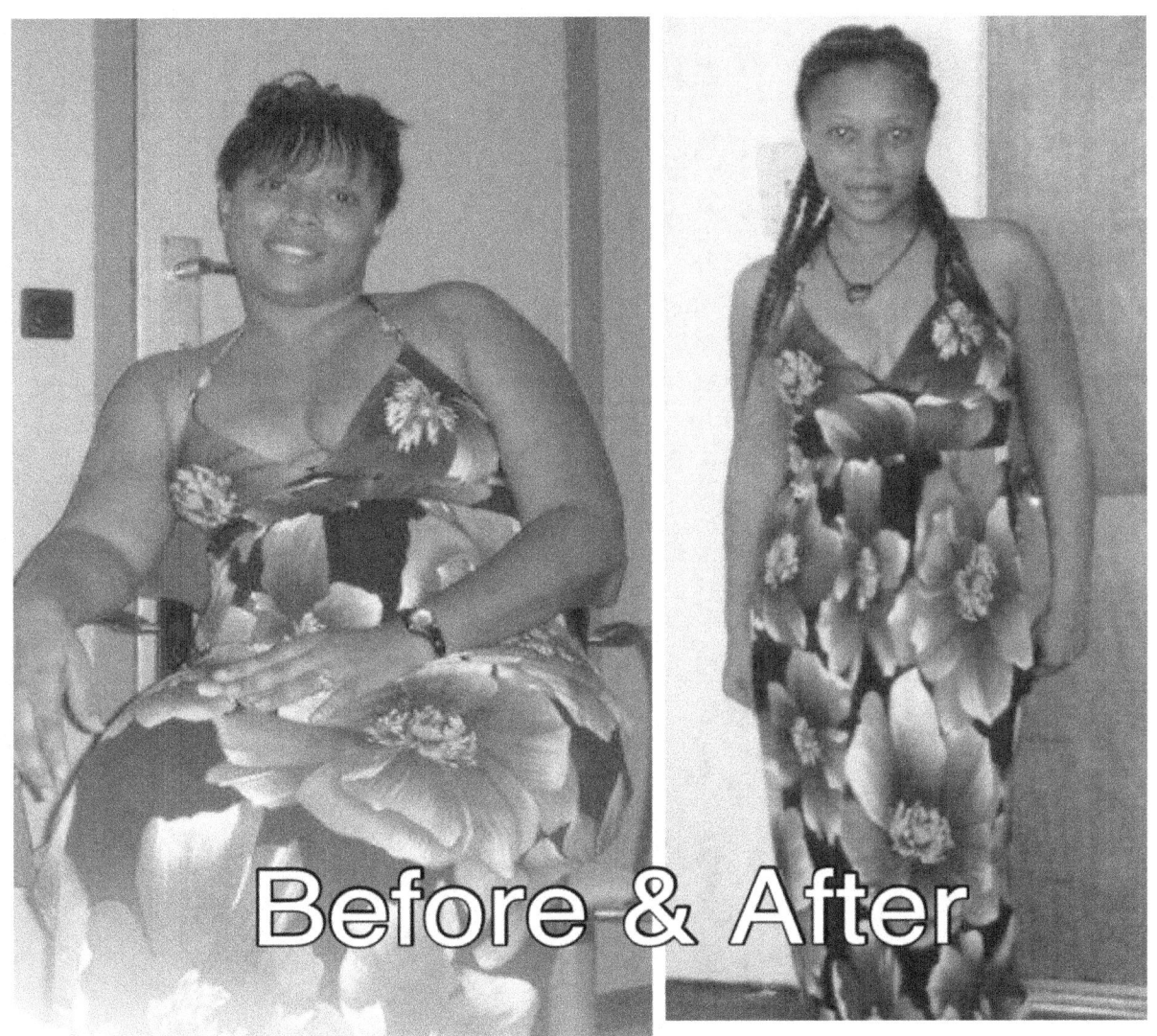

Before & After

2010 Feb.                                            2012 Feb.

What a difference a year can make when you make a difference

What if I never made the change, I do not even want to imagine where I would be at now, or how I would look. Wow.

Before                    After

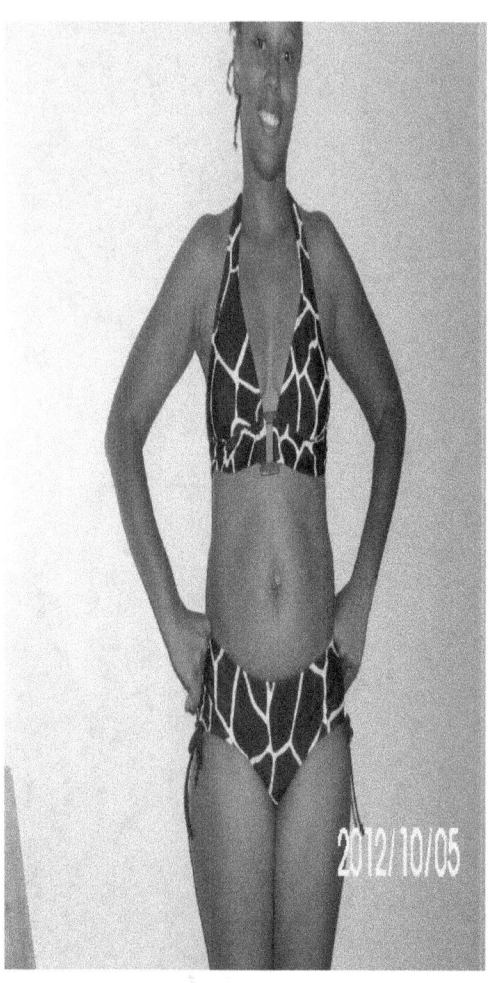 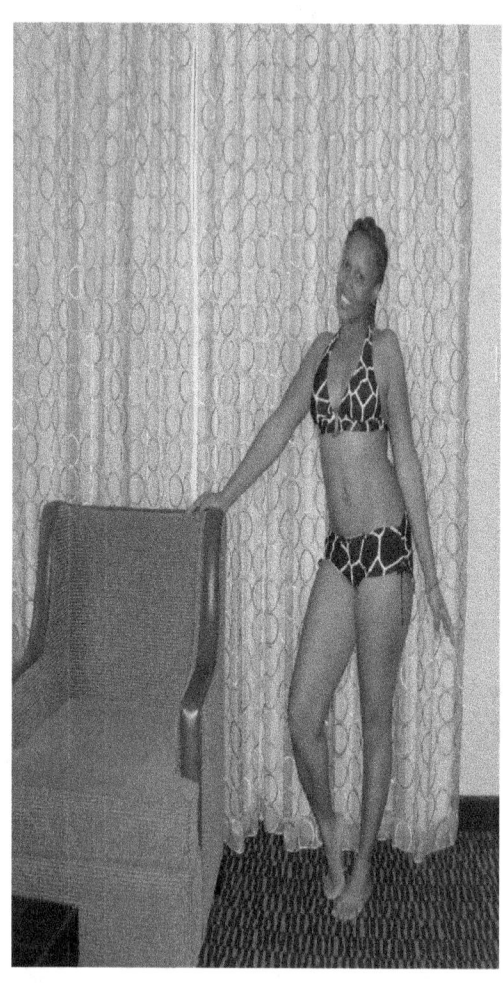

I was pleased with the first pic because I still looked a lot better
than I had 2 years before but now this one is even better.
Progress is everything.

I was on my gym grind and loving it... fitting into pants I could not fit before.

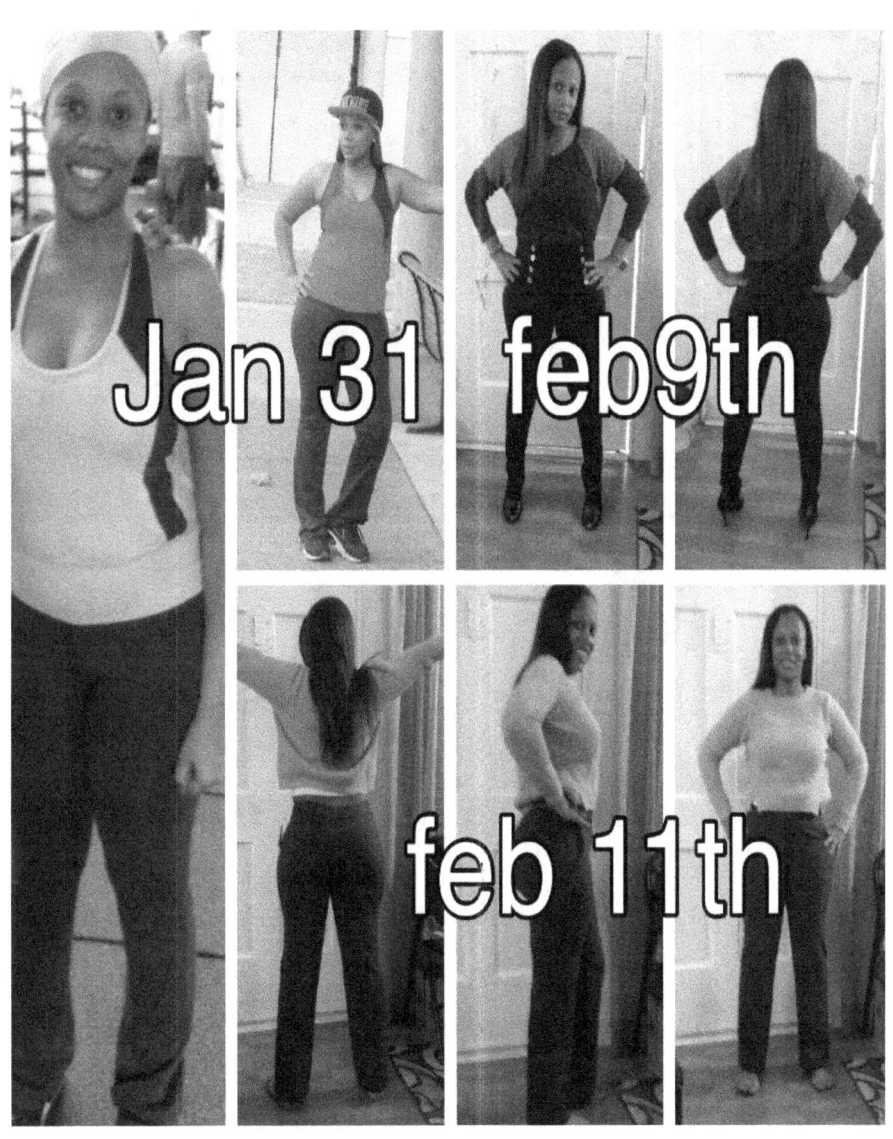

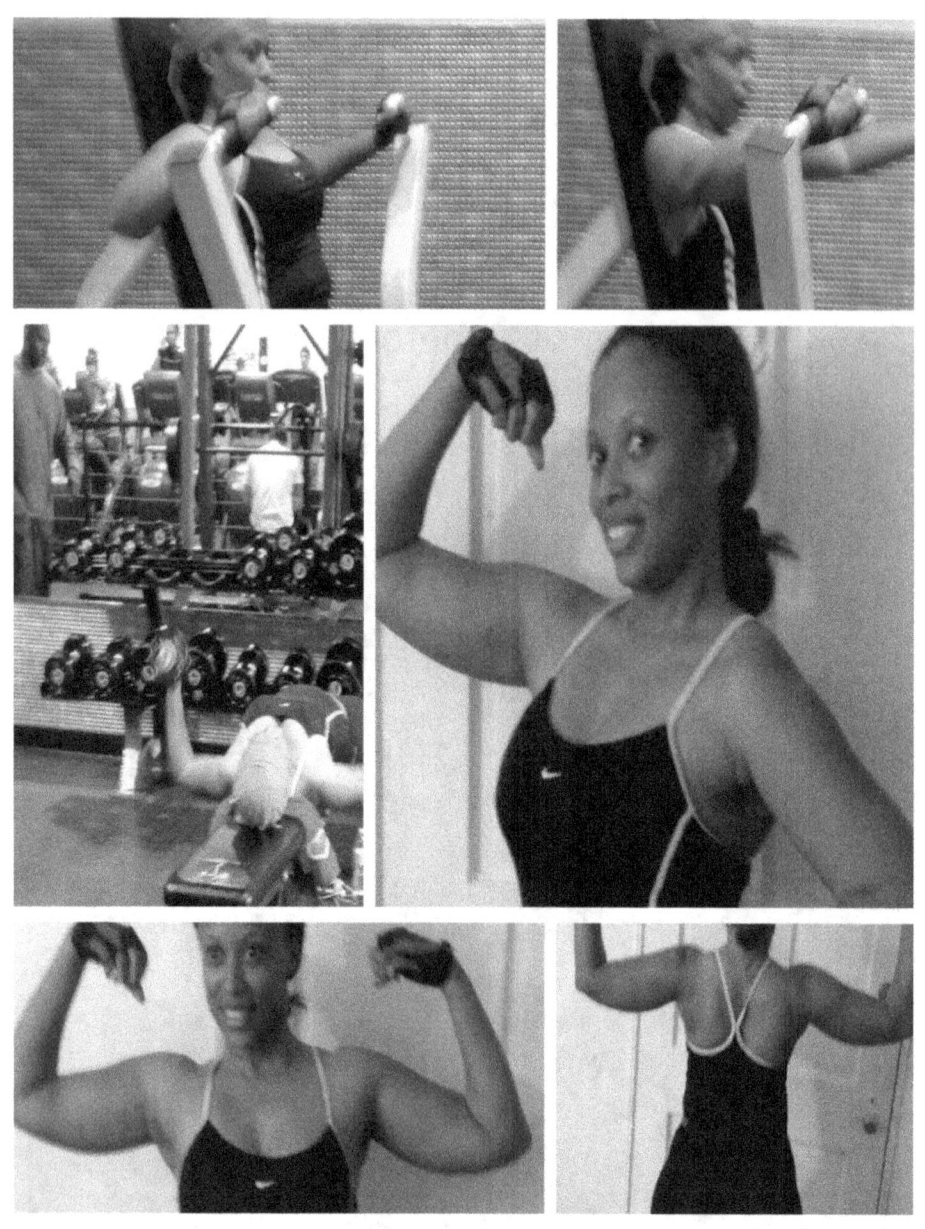

Enjoying my guns but kept them down so I would still look feminine.

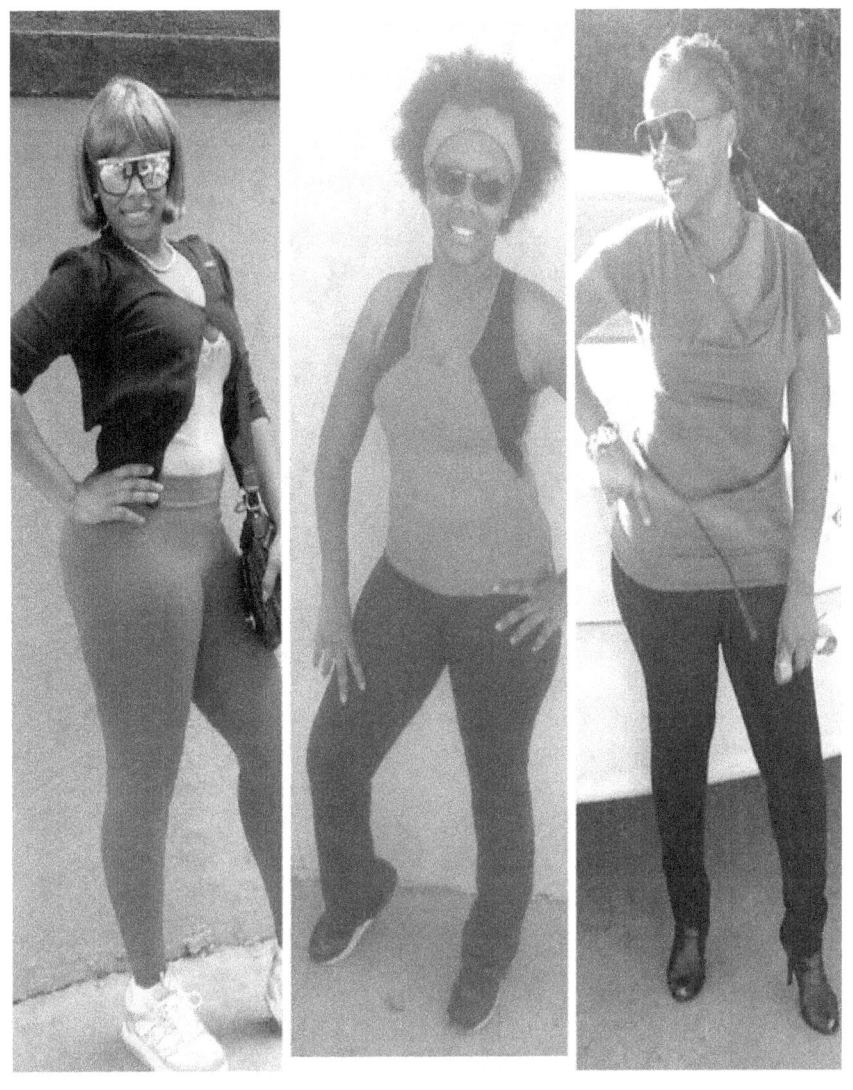

I love these pics; they were all taken at great moments and times in my life.  Memories to look back on and smile.

Feb. 2012

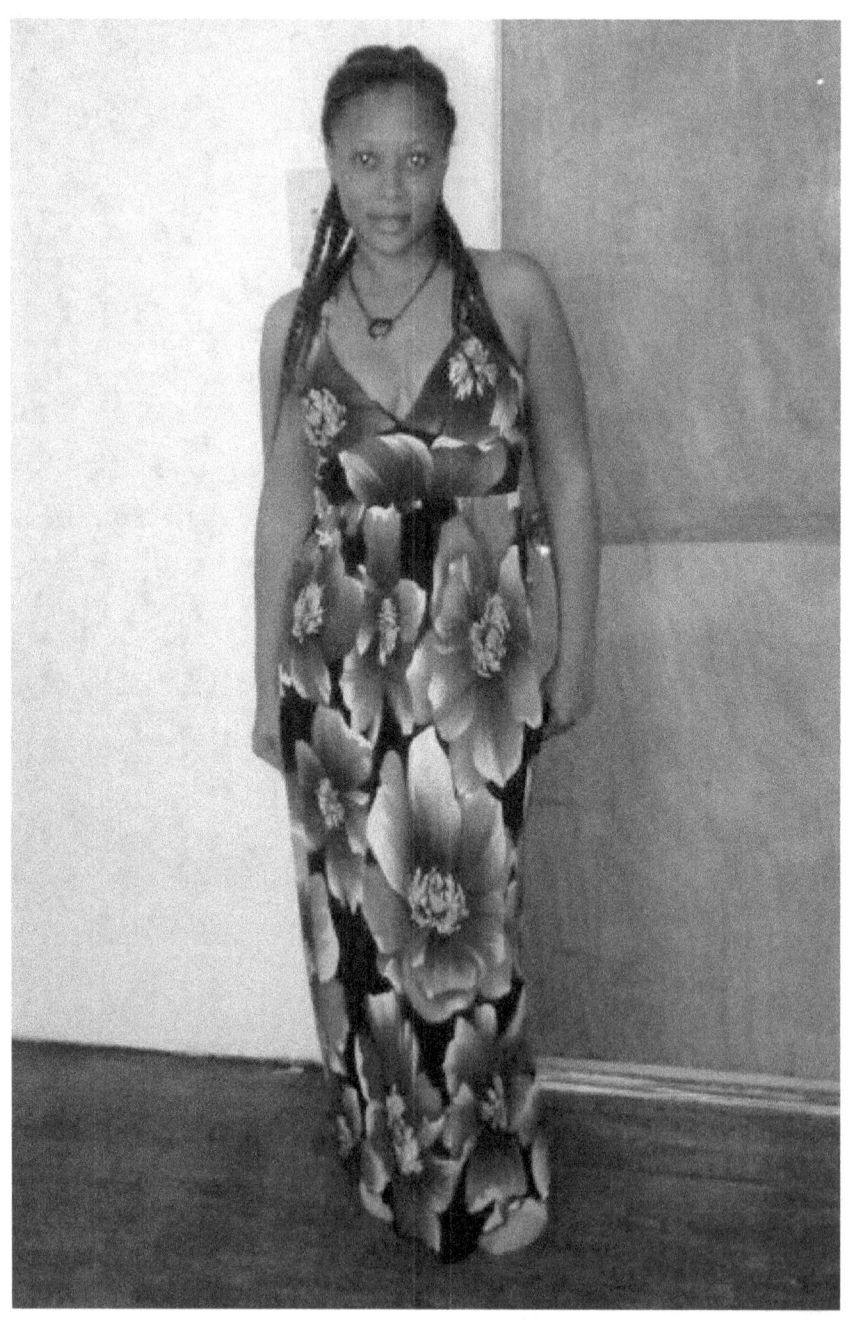

I was so pleased to take this after pic, the before was a woman I did not even know, she was someone I was not pleased with and completely needed to change.

Wala a brand new me!!!

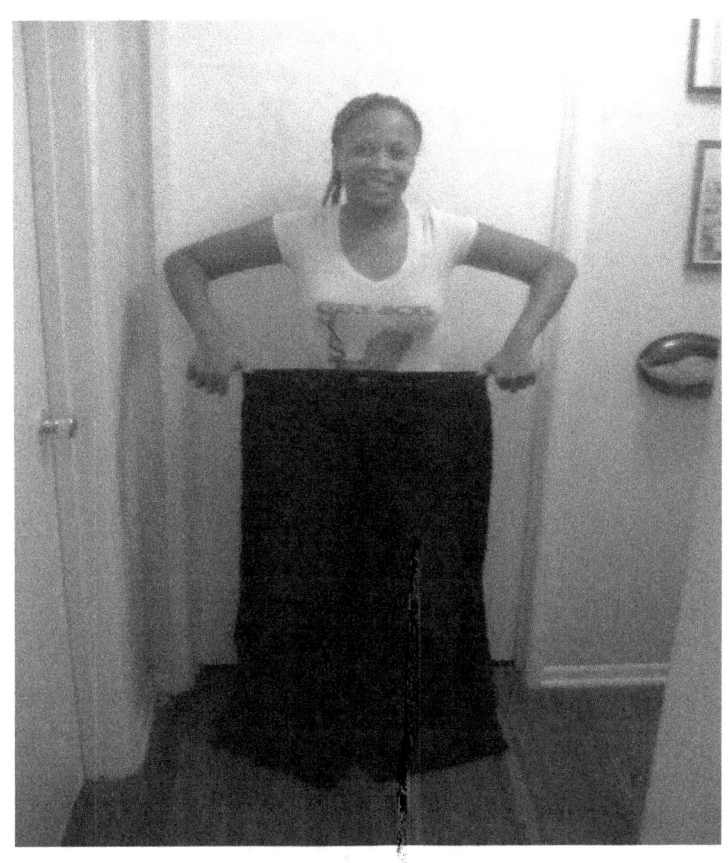

No more size 16 and 18 or 20's

I love this pic looking back now I cannot believe I fit those pants
at one time. Wow, thank God for change!

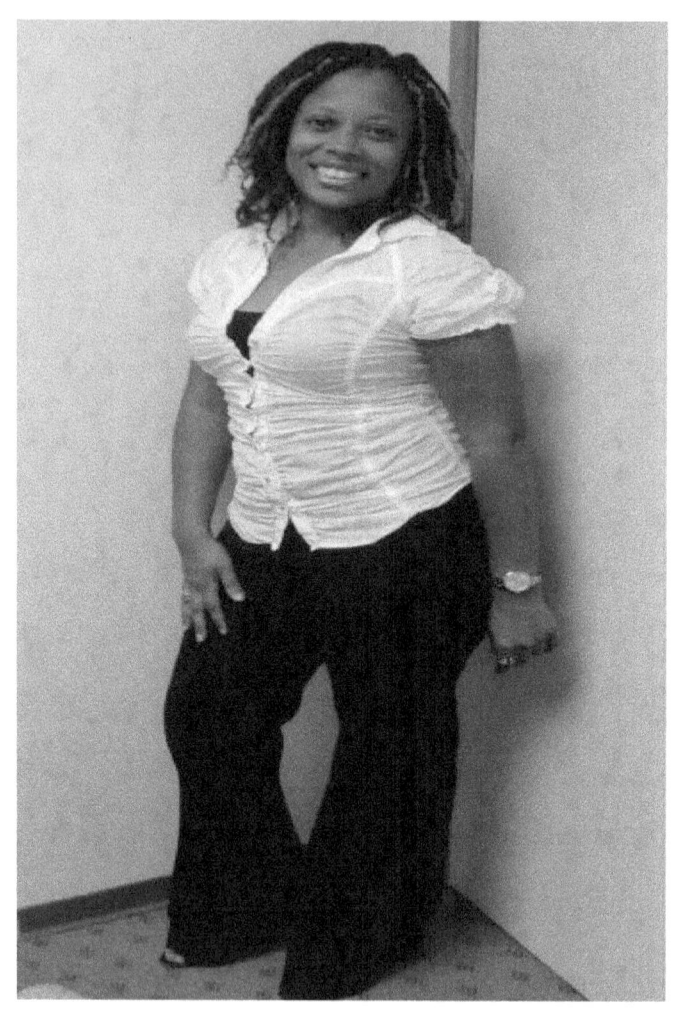

I was happy here, I can remember this day like yesterday right after my weight lost and I had on some new pants that fit great.

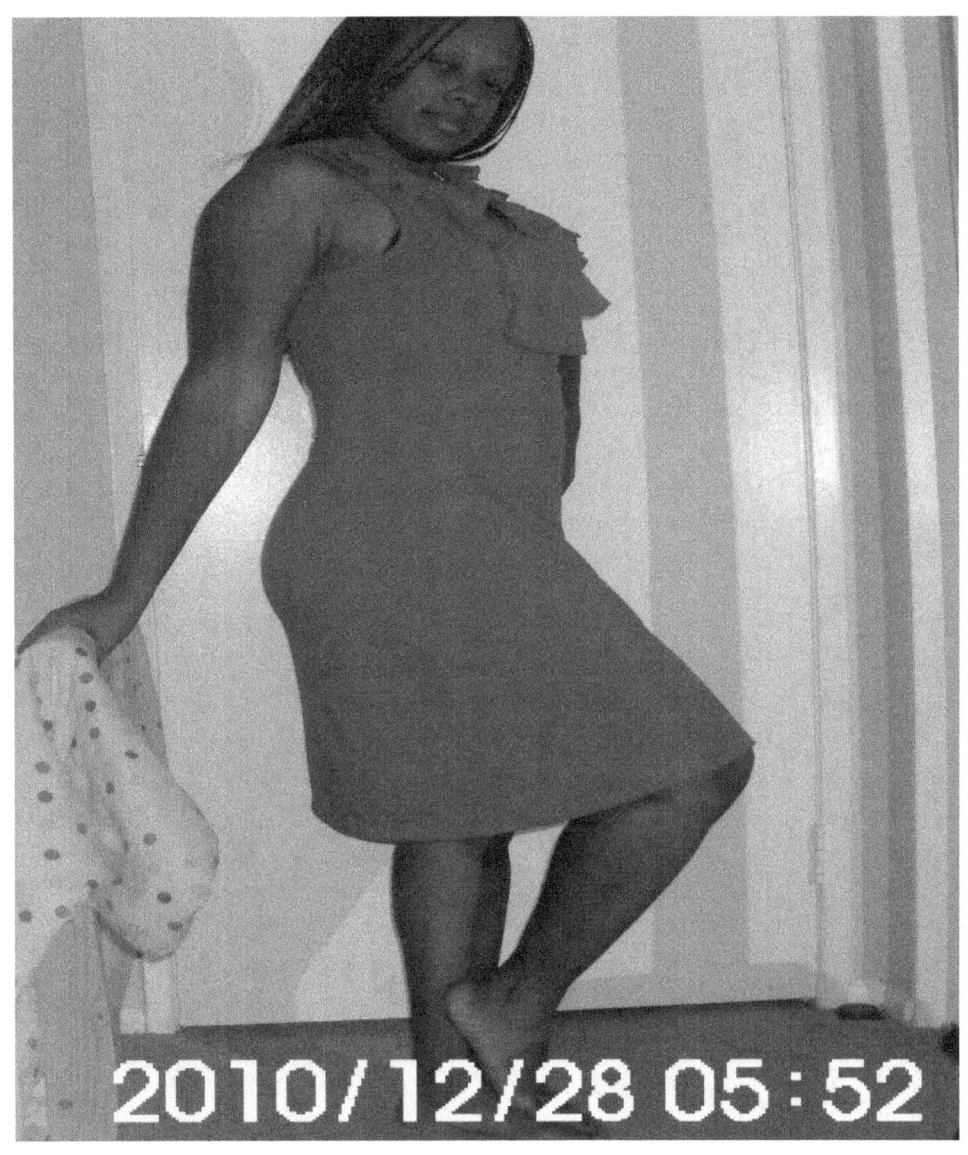

2010/12/28 05:52

On page 38 the before pic in the same dress

Well this is the body I wanted to see in the dress when I bought it, imagine that, I fit my motivation dress well now.

I hope these pictures are inspiring you to change. Like I said no one says you must be a size 2 or 4 or even 10 but be the best that you are and do something different and take pics throughout the journey so you can see and show others your progress.

None of these are edited or tampered with, these are all real pics and telling the story of my life. I hope it helps you and motivates you to tell your story too. If you do not have one to tell, just make the start.  You too can have the same happy ending.

# MORE AFTER PICS- from 2011 until the present

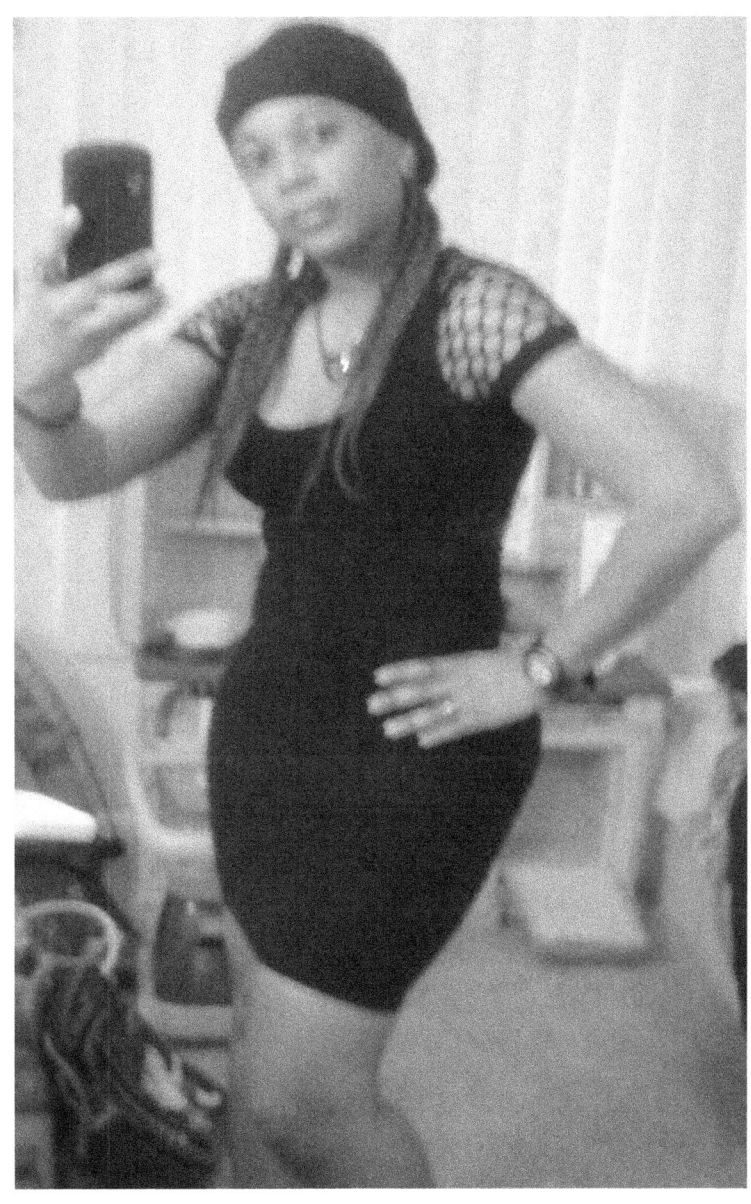

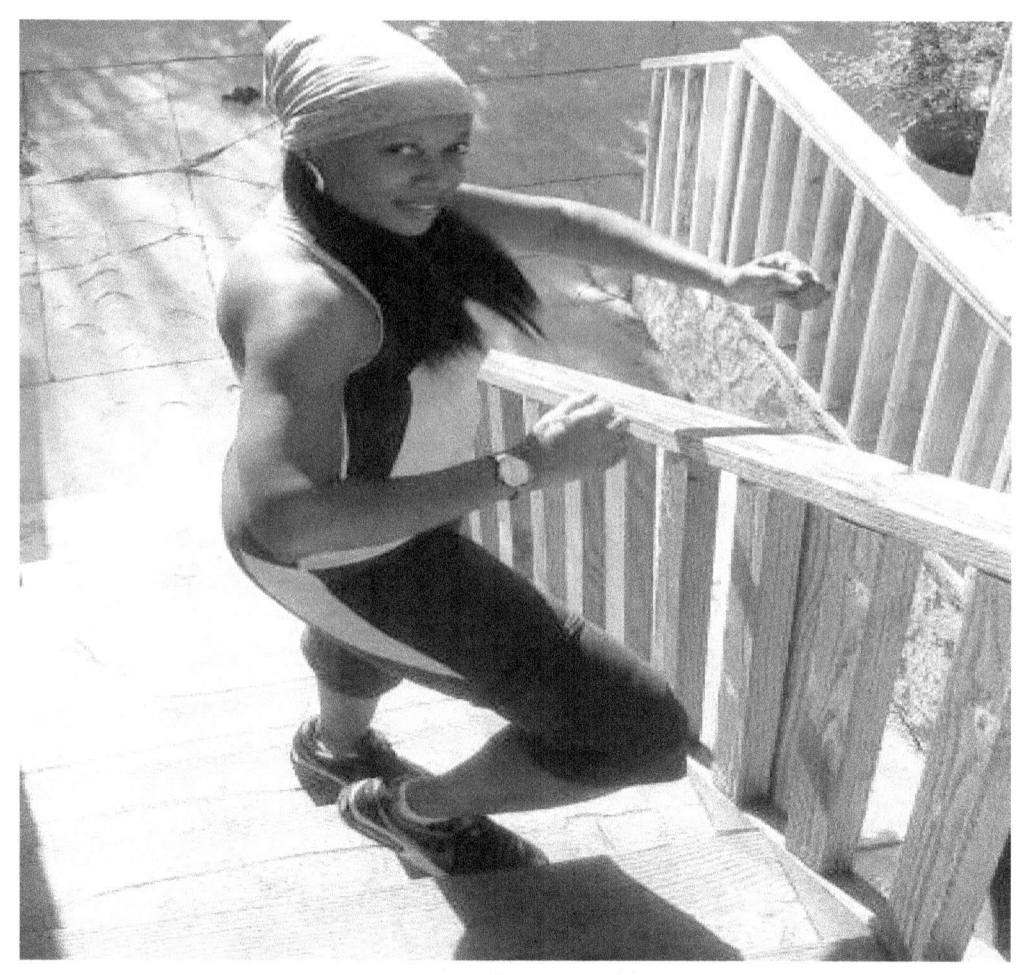

Awe shucks, I Loved this time I was doing well and had just got back in touch with a good friend who is now my fiancé. ☺

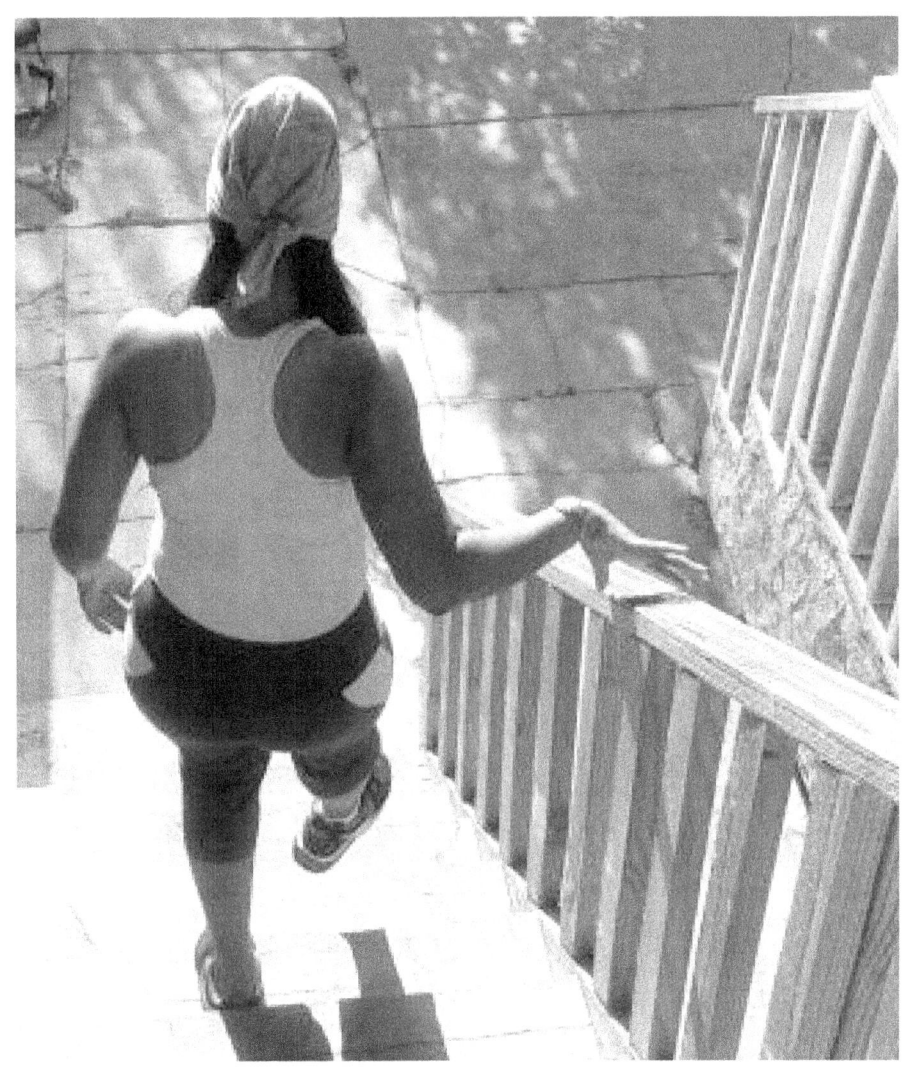

He took these two shots for me and captured a time of great
joy and restoration for me.

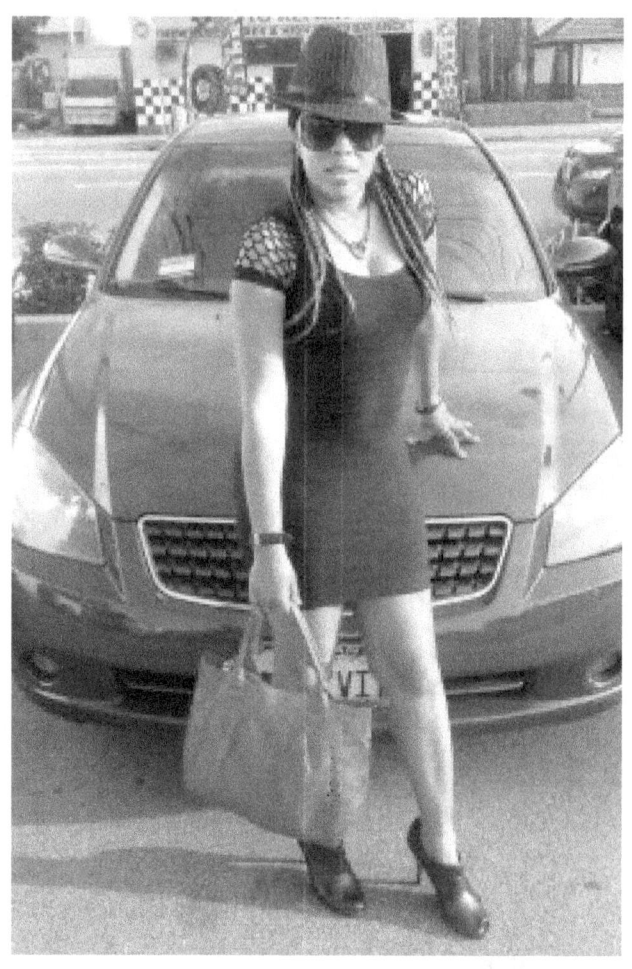

Went to eat out with my friend- now fiancé I never dreamt I could fit that type of dress during my big days.

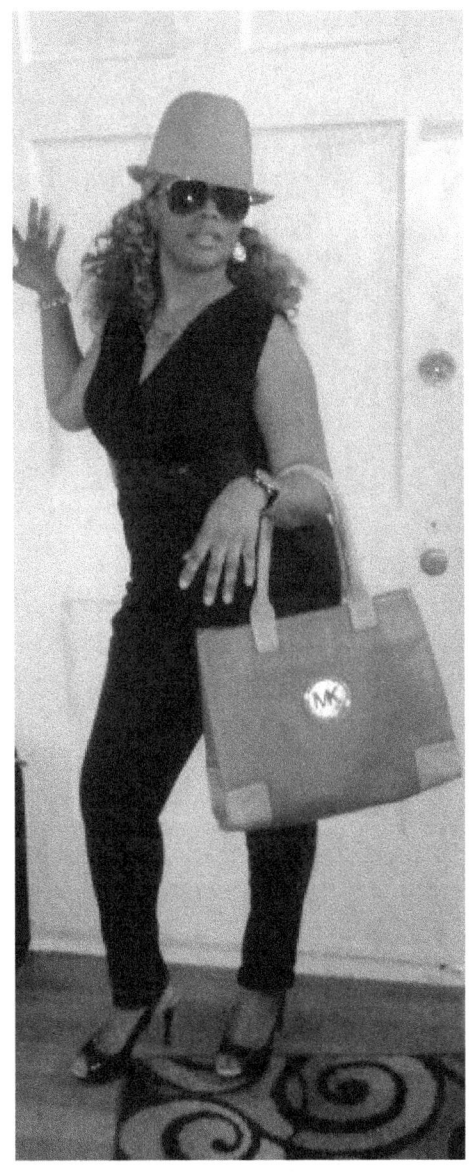

I was too much ha, but loving being who I was meant to be

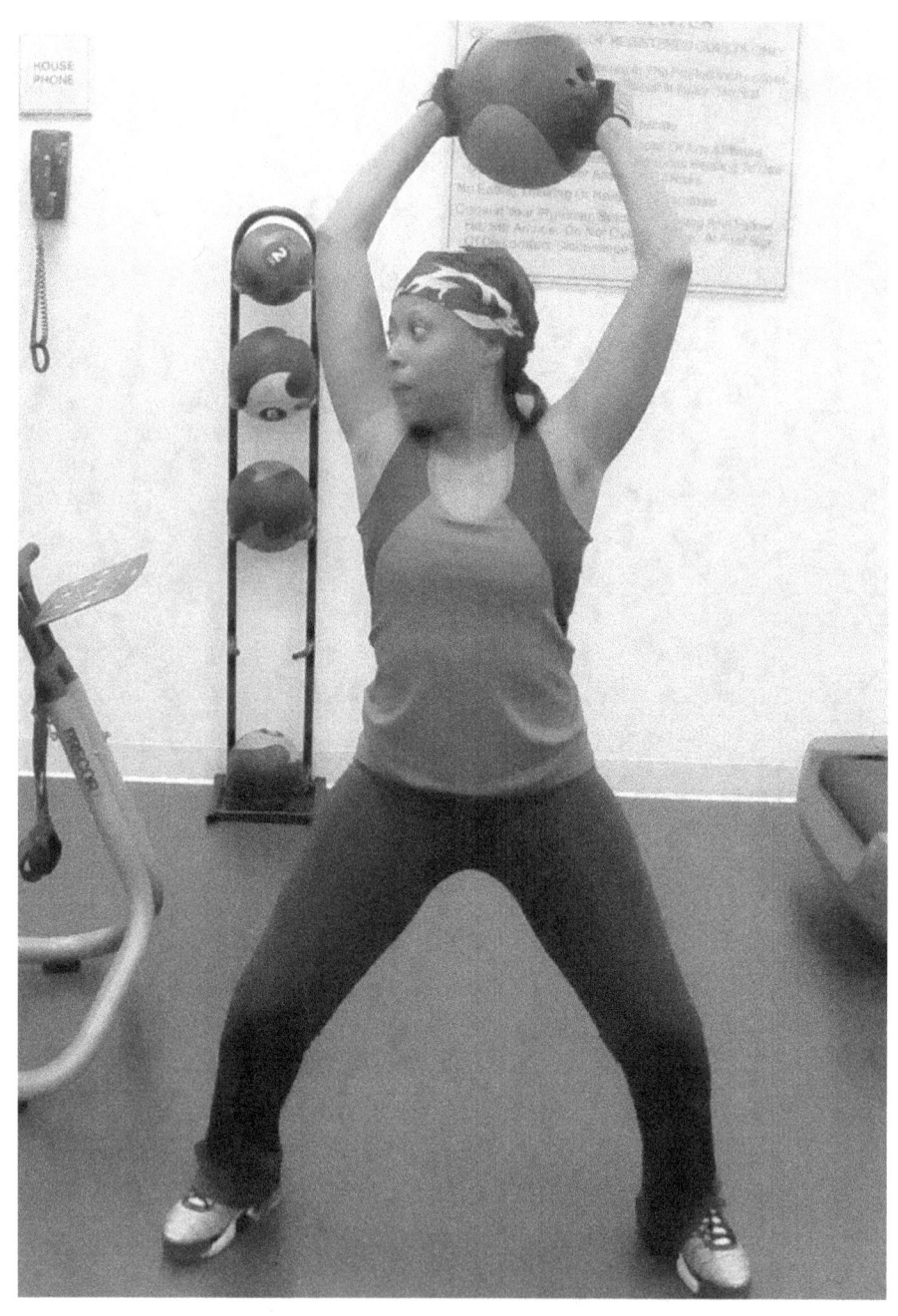

Doing what I loved, exercising

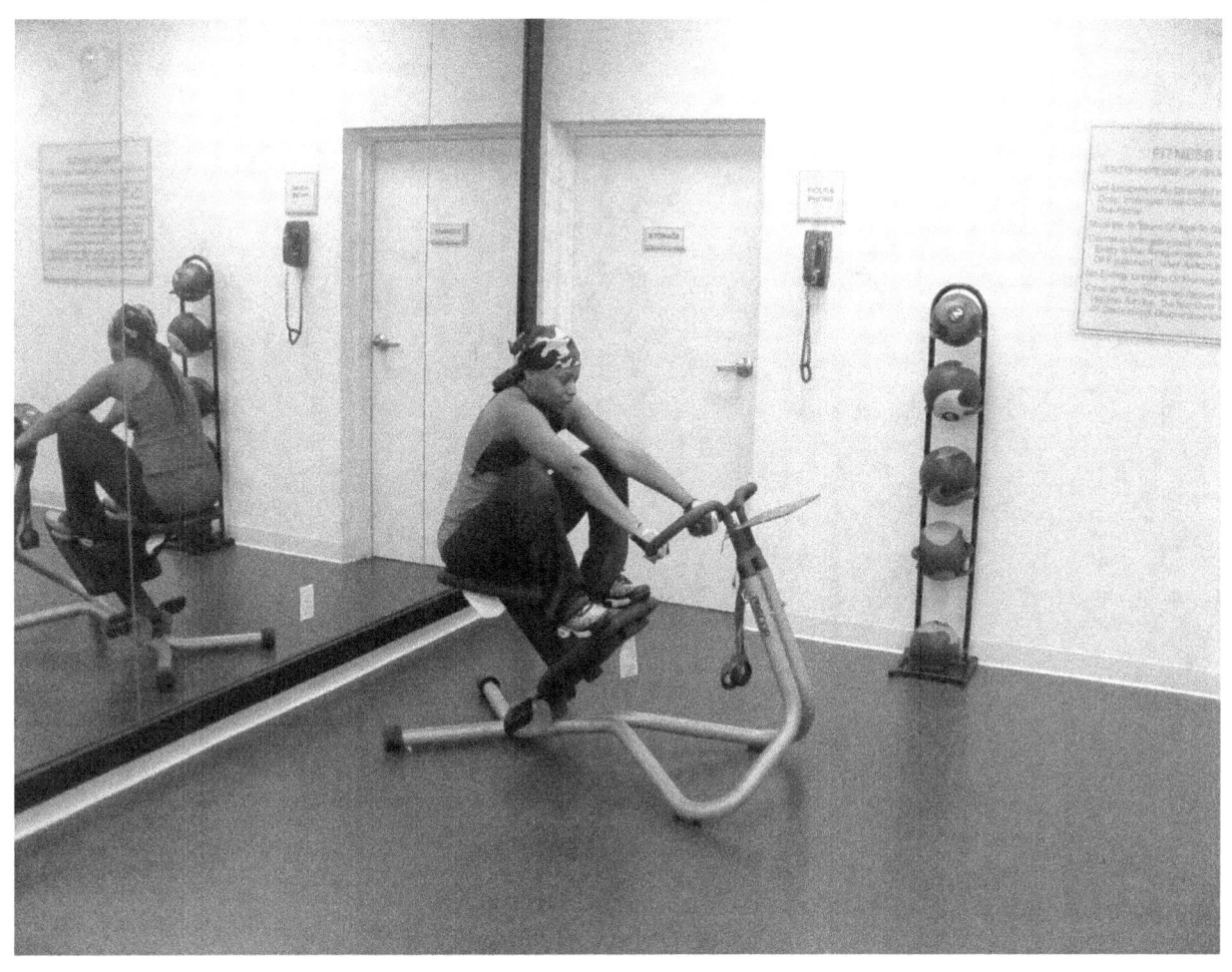

I still cannot seem to figure this one out haa.

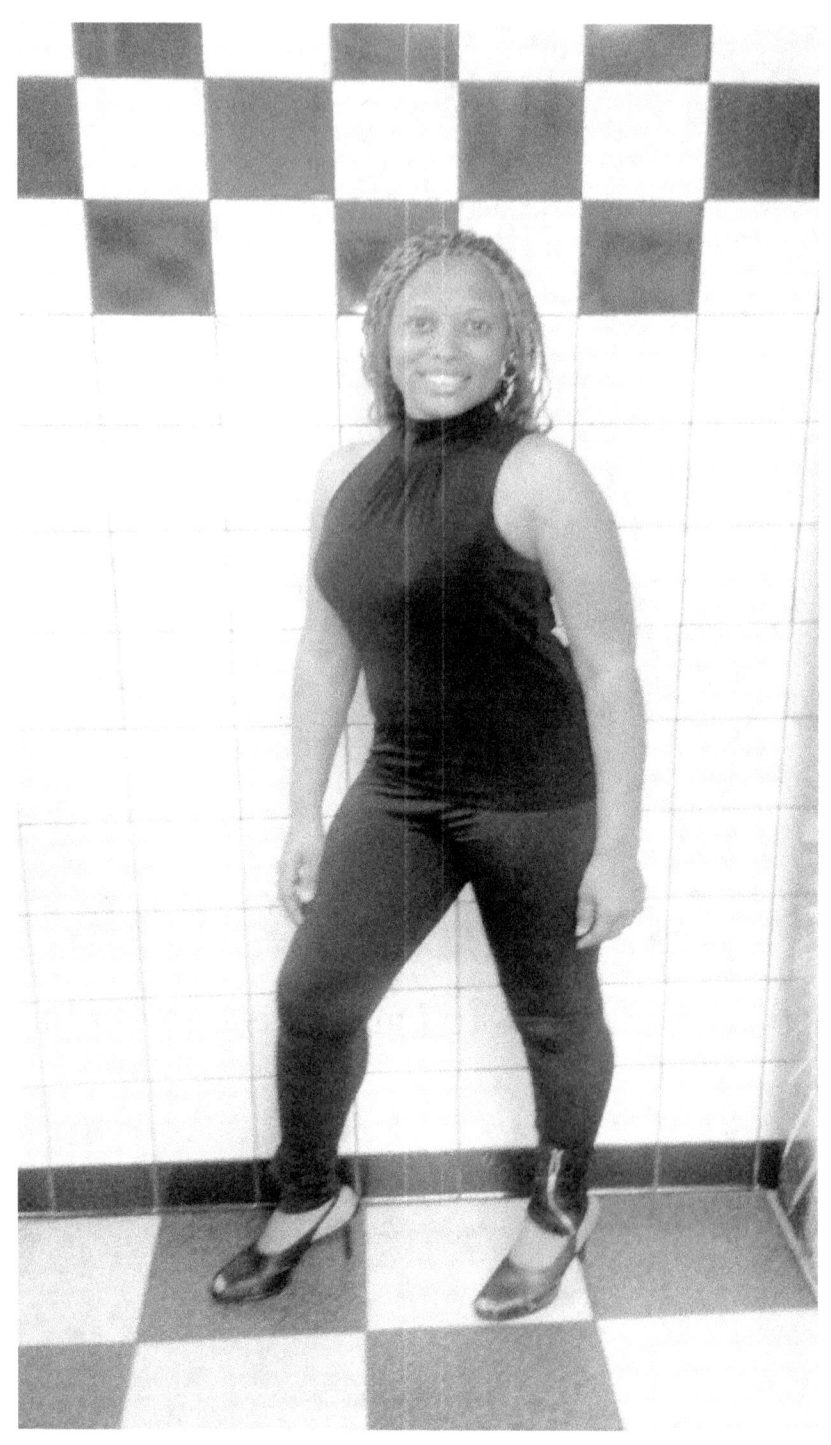

Well, I was on my way out and was loving the fact that I was fit and happy.

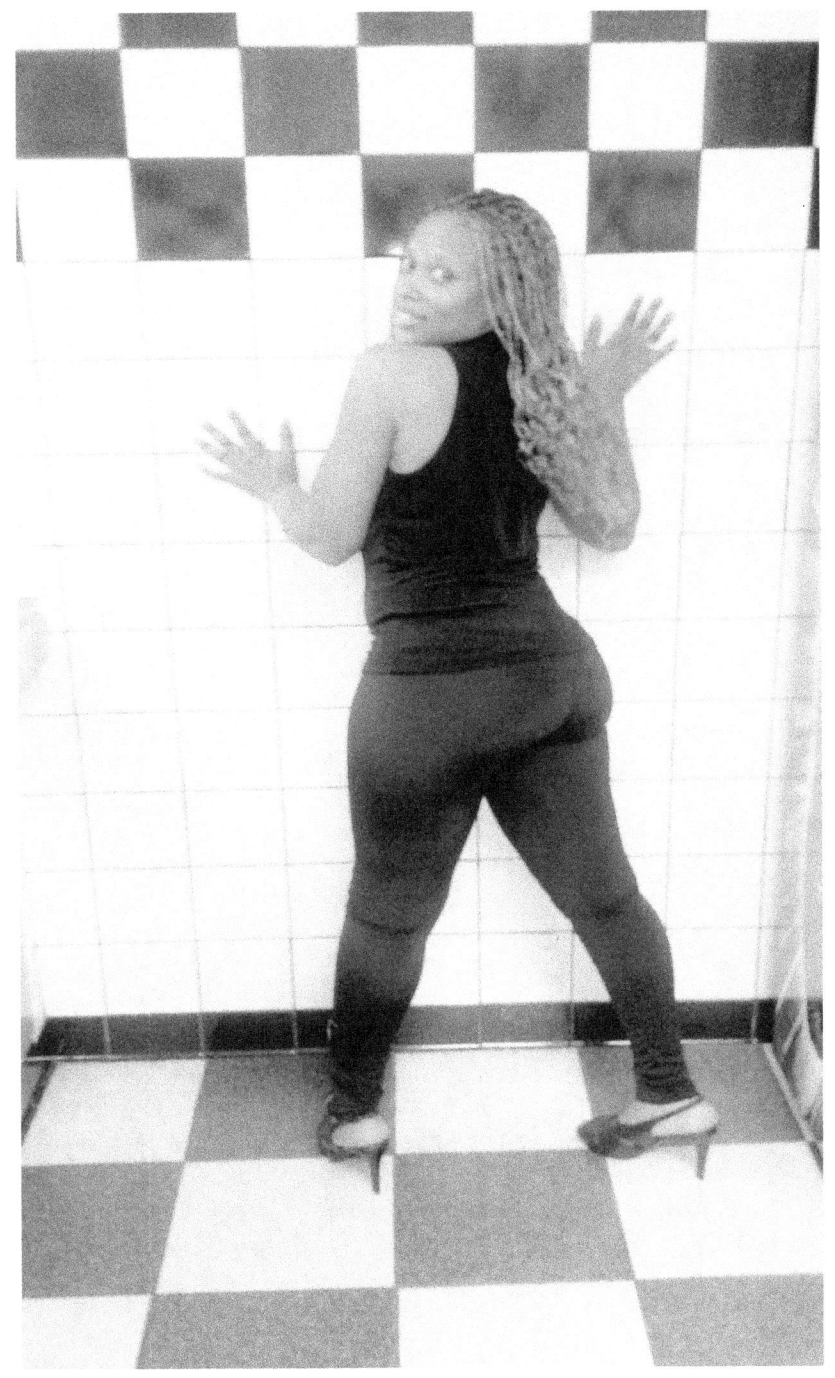

Always had to have a back-shot ha when you lose weight you love every angel.

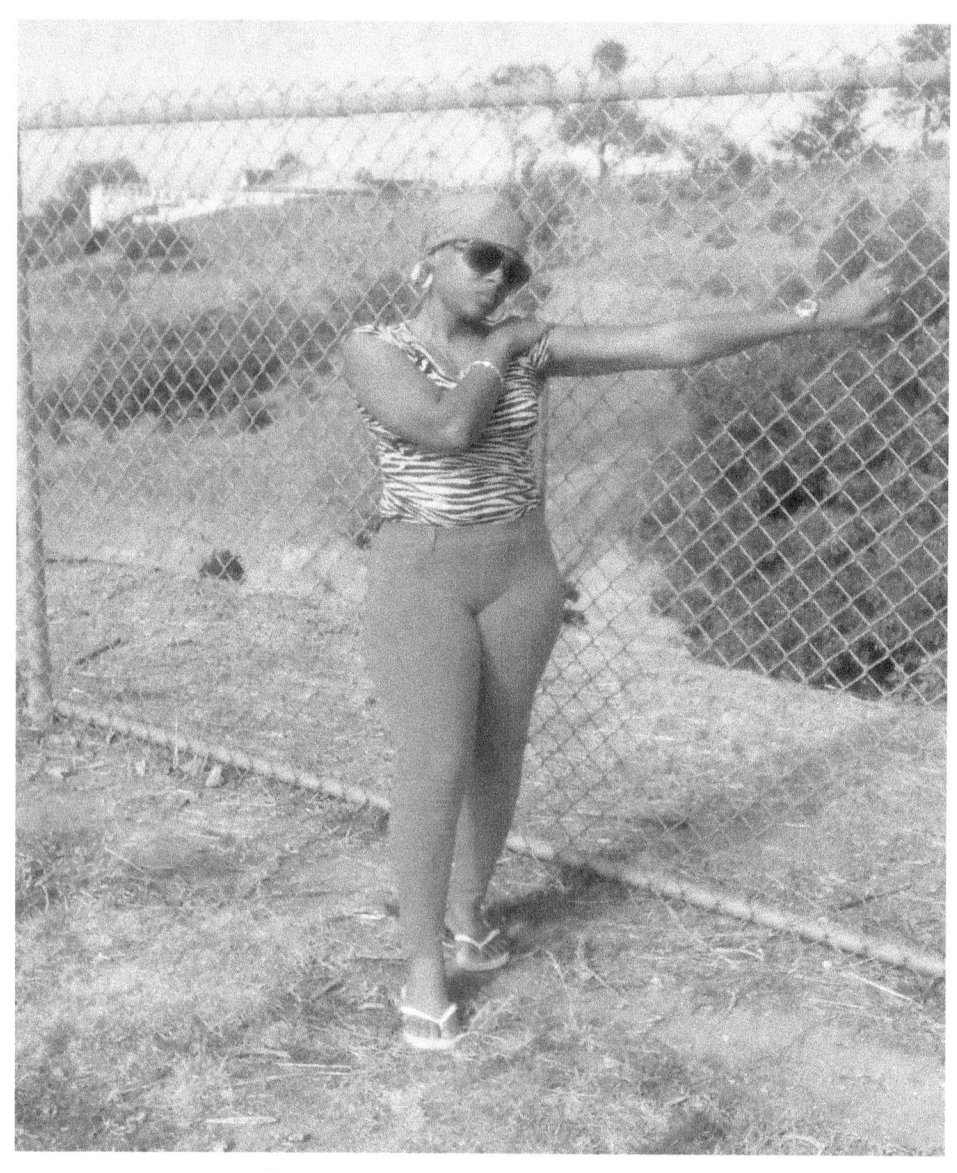

I was reflecting on how much peace I had in my life then

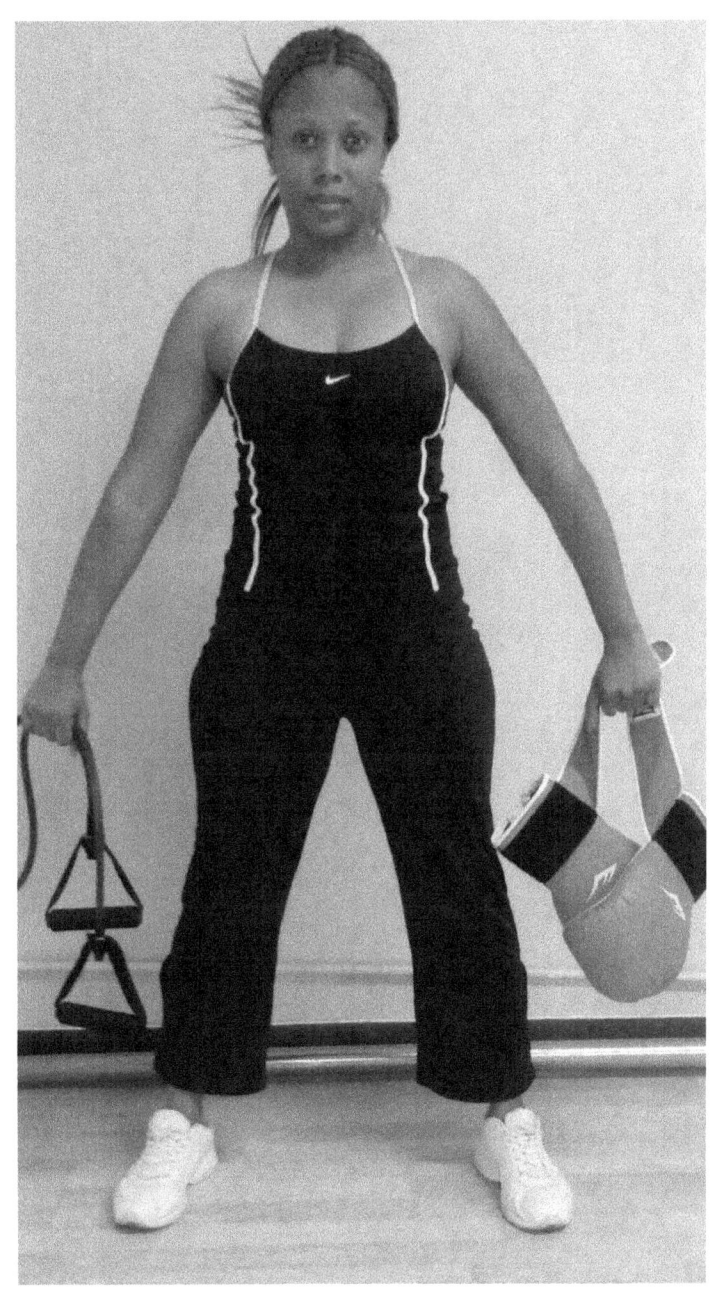

During the time, I was working with one of my coaches learning more techniques and life lessons to keep me going strong

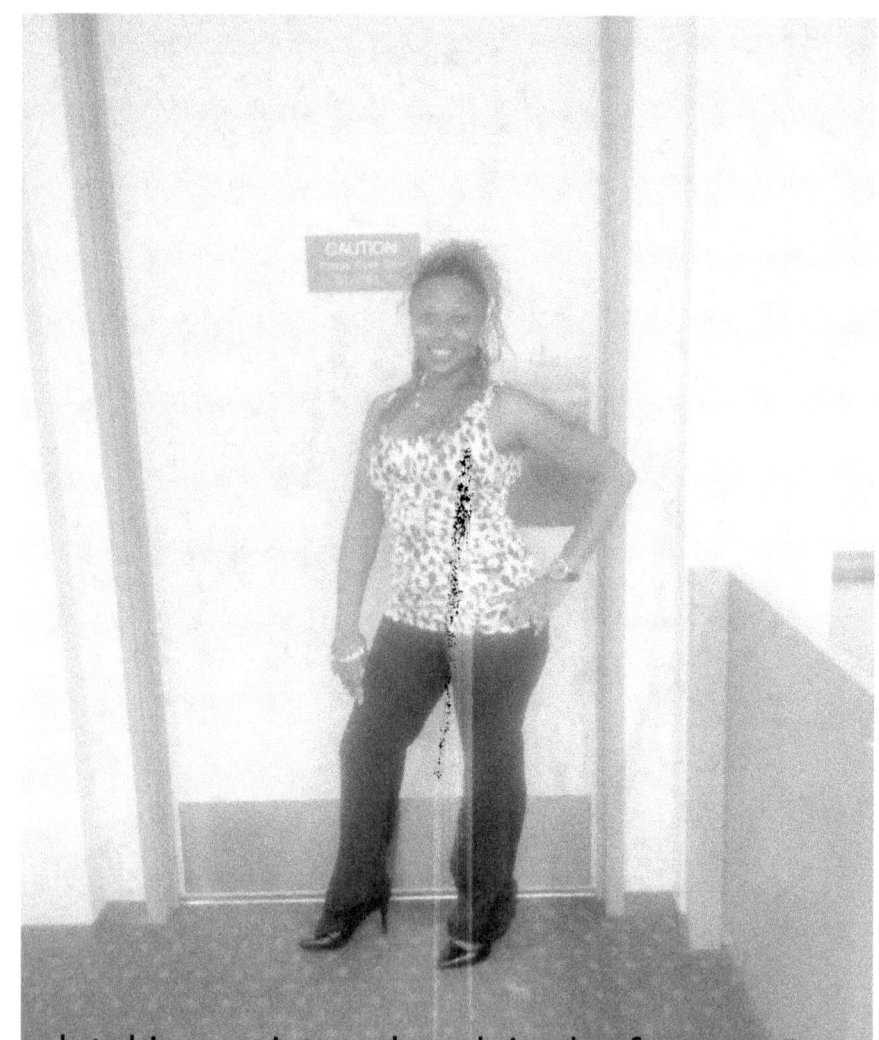

At work taking a picture break in the famous Dept. 401

At County, wide fitness walk

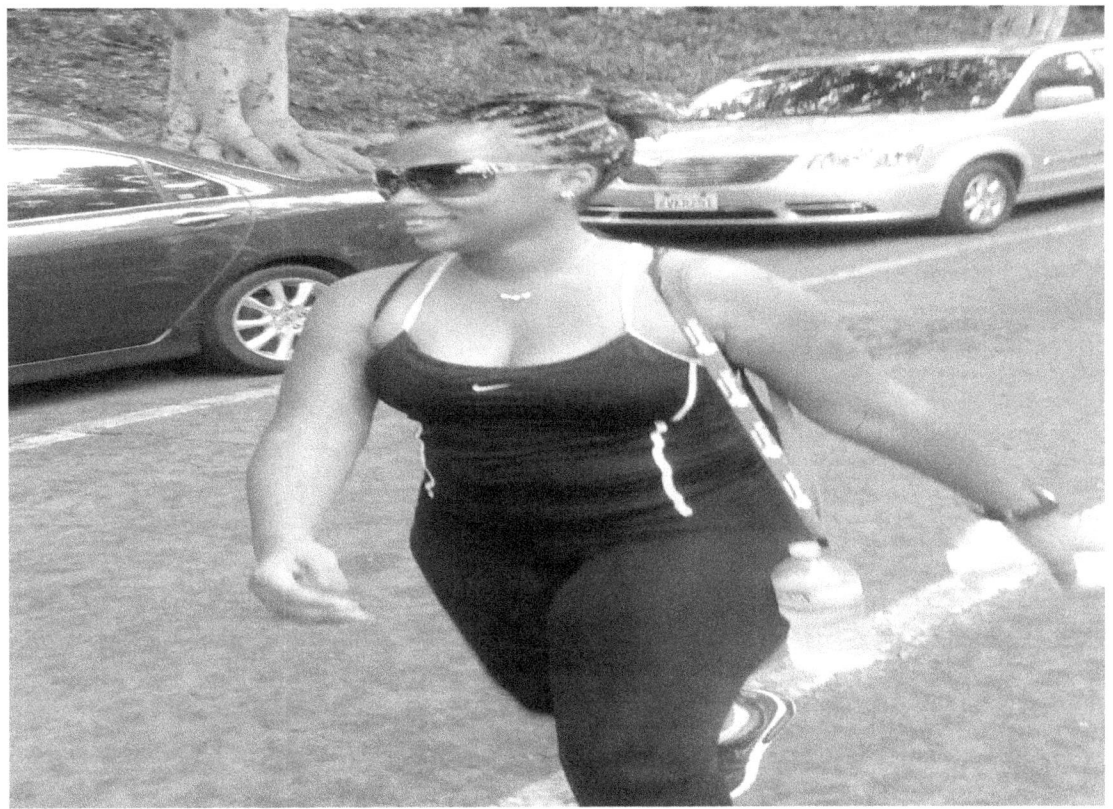

I loved being a part of these fitness days so much fun

# LOVING THE BODY, I AM IN! ☺

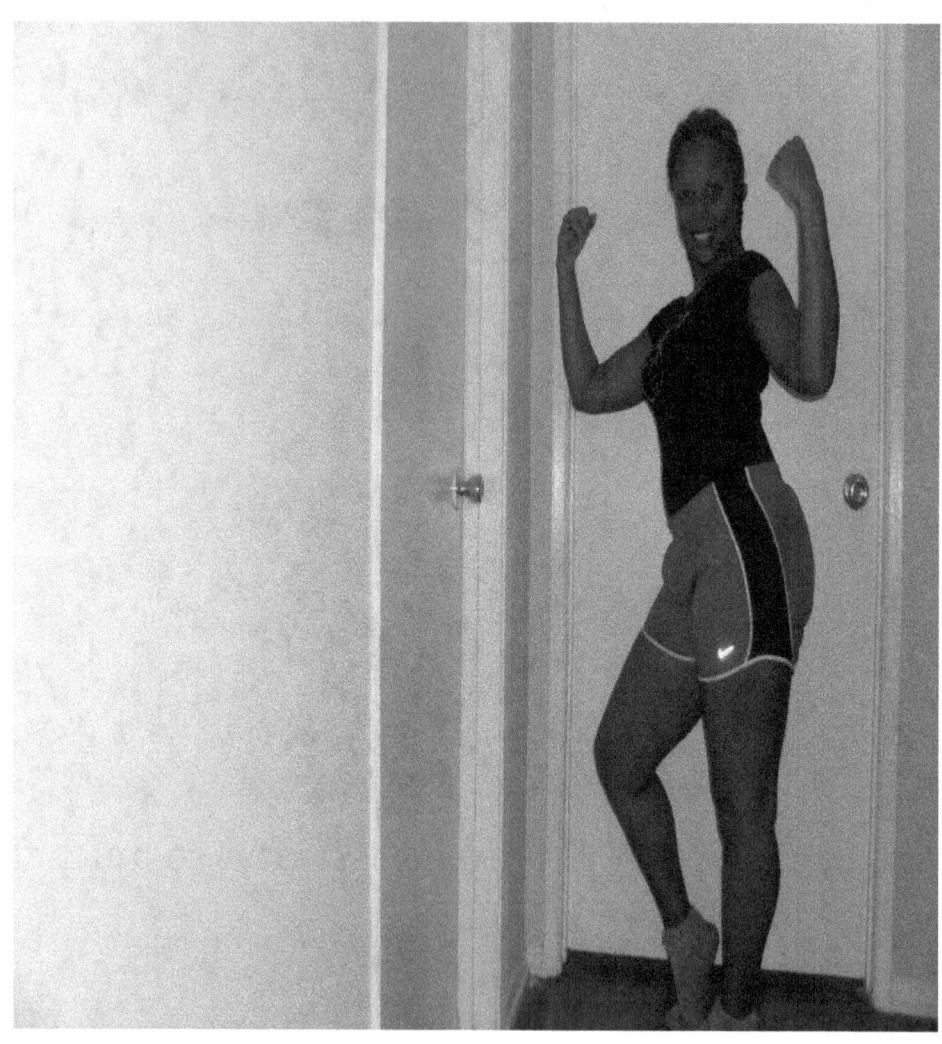

At my son's dedication service, I was back to my old self again

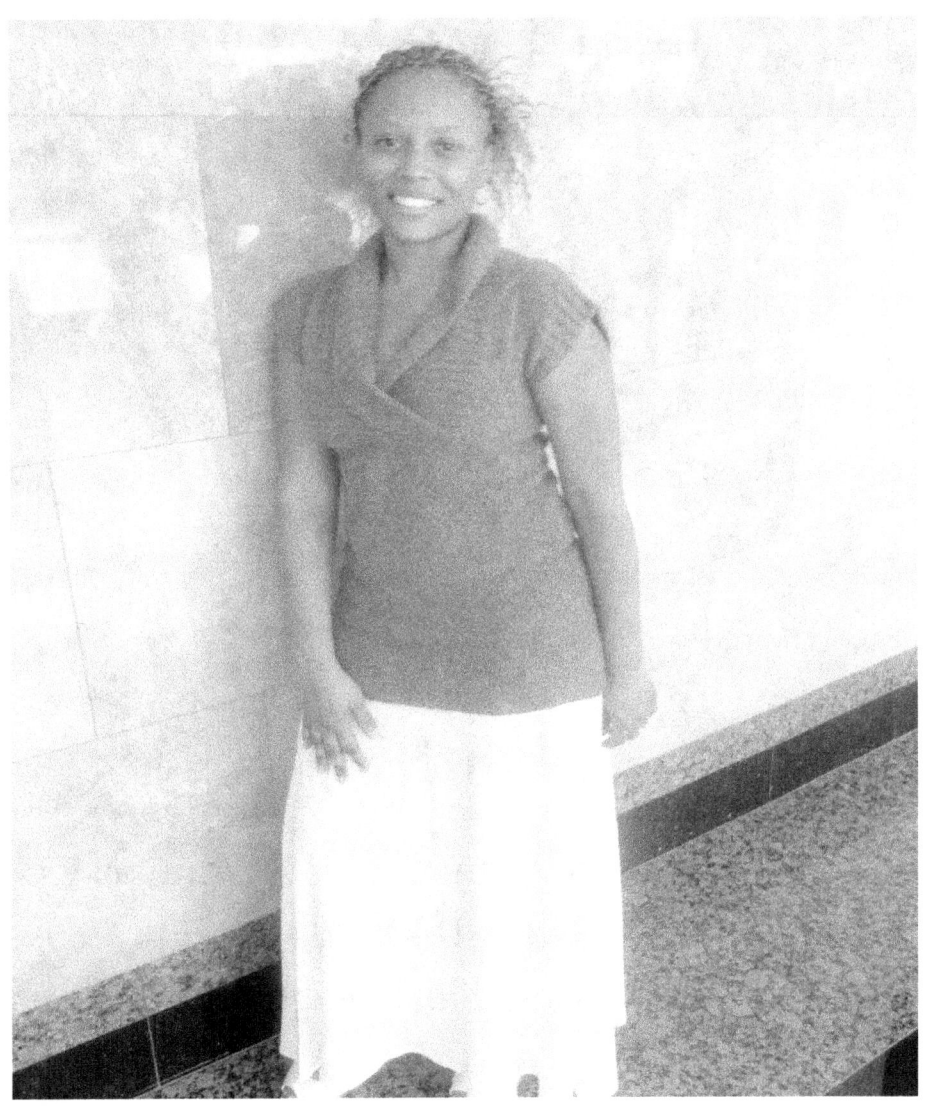

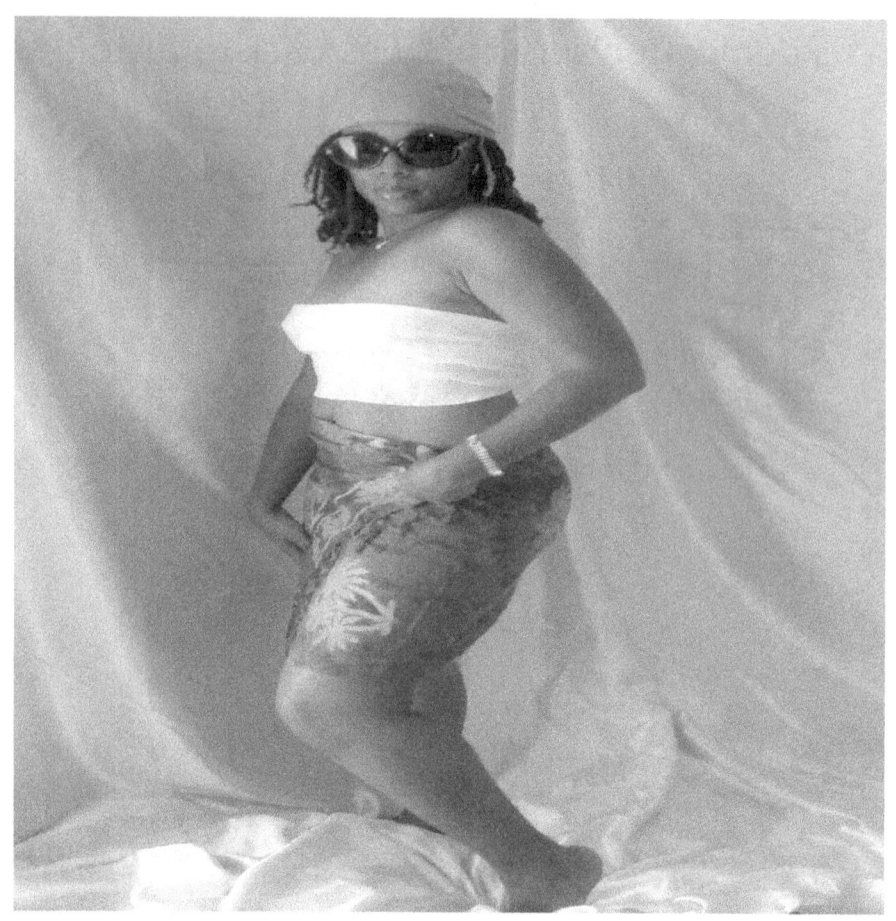

My boyfriend then- now fiancé took this one ha we love photoshoots and this one was great... when you can use a head wrap as a blouse you know you lost weight ha, and a scarf for a skirt. Look like I'm ready for the islands.

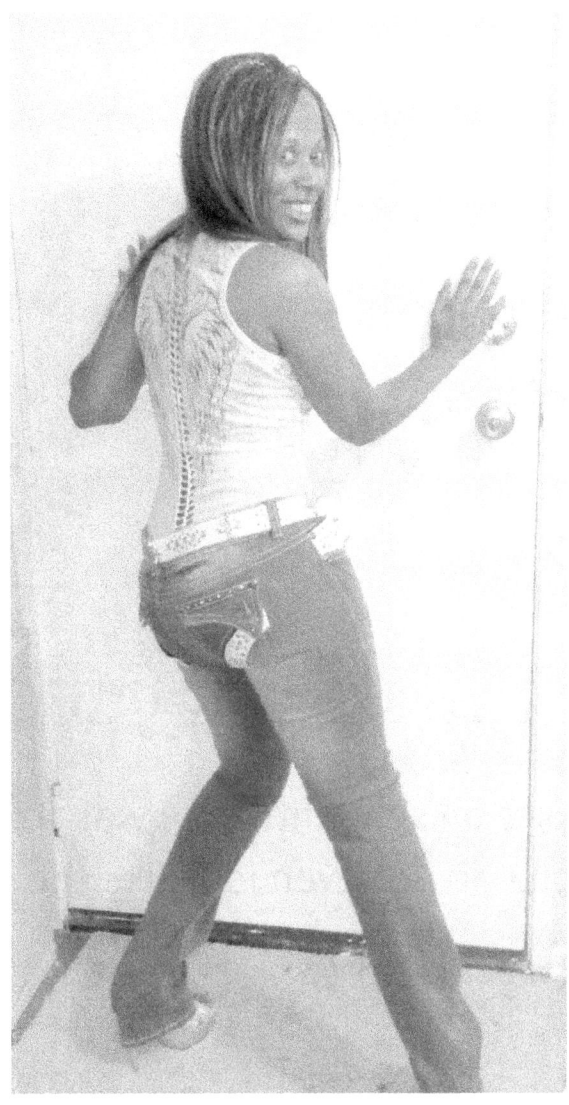

Birthday party time- June of 2011

Talk about being happy I was excited about this time in life: I was fit, trim, ready to party and my hair was on point thanks to my cousin Porche-beautician extraordinaire.

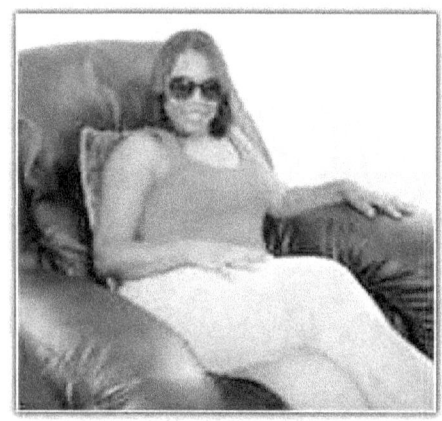
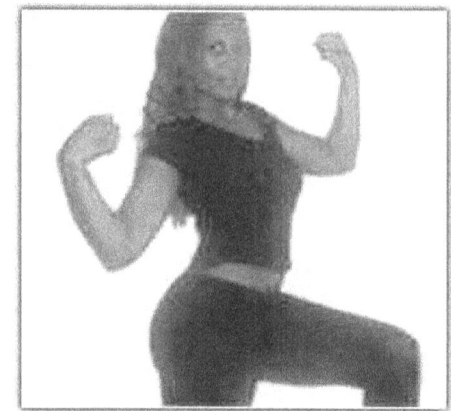

**BEFORE**        **AFTER**

## LockMarie Lost 65 Pounds!

I shared these pics on shapefit.com I was so excited for this transformation I do not even look like the same person.

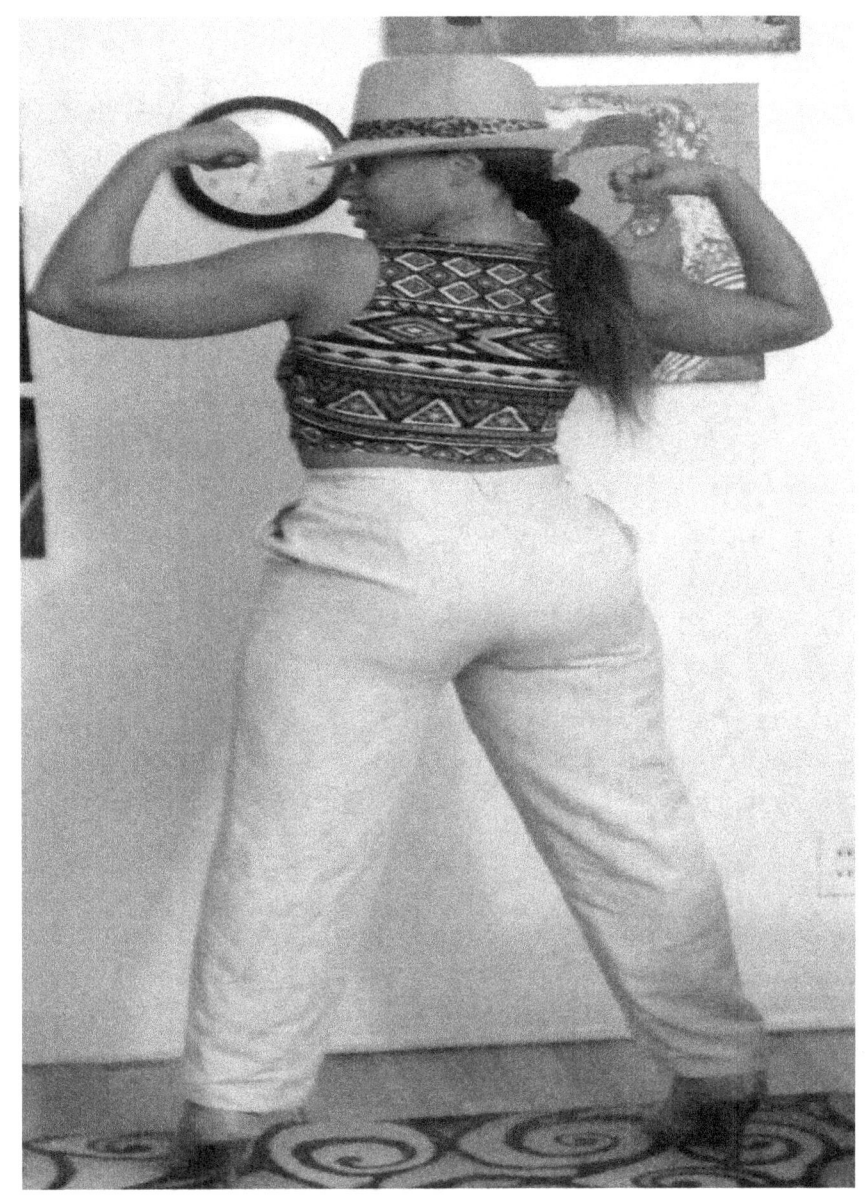

I was so pumped to fit this outfit ha like for real

Another great fitness event. I was so excited to be there. Wow, my arms were normal sizes again. Great achievement!!!

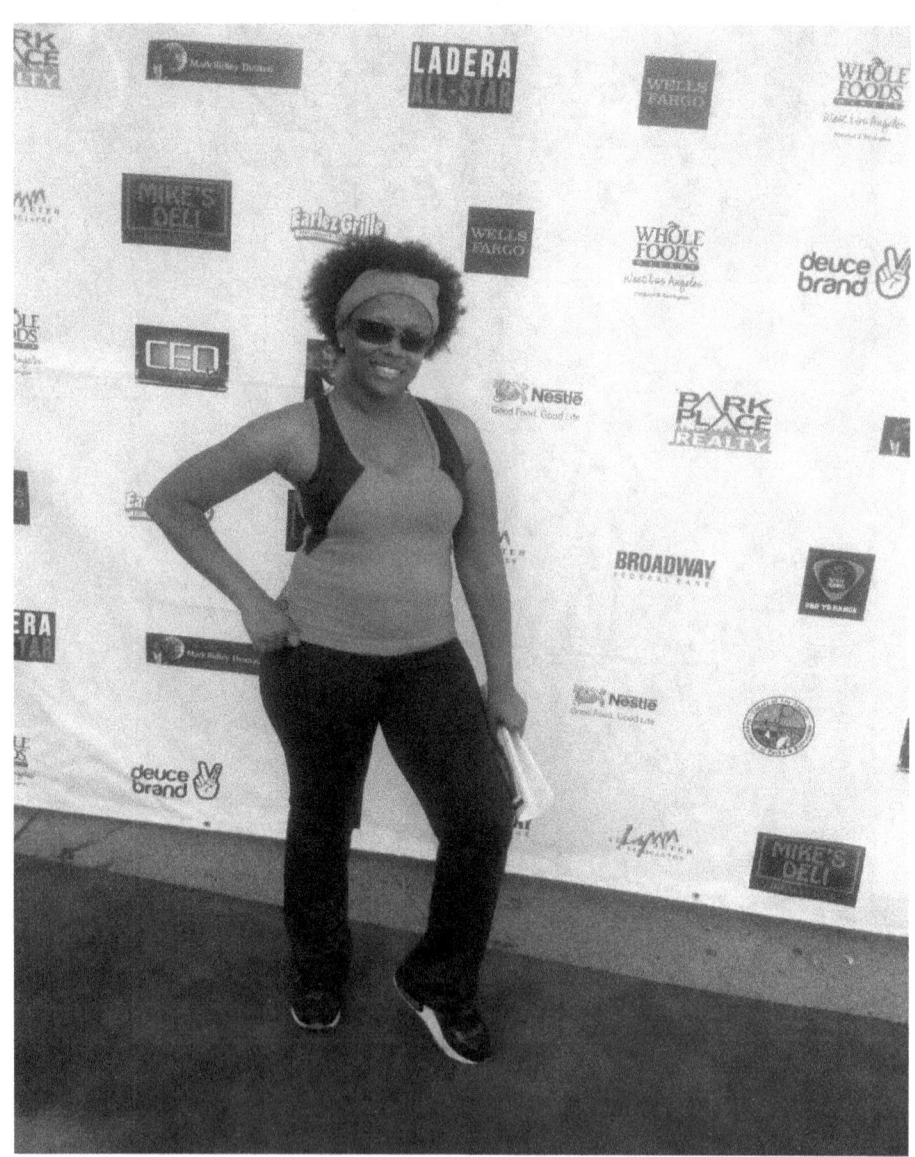

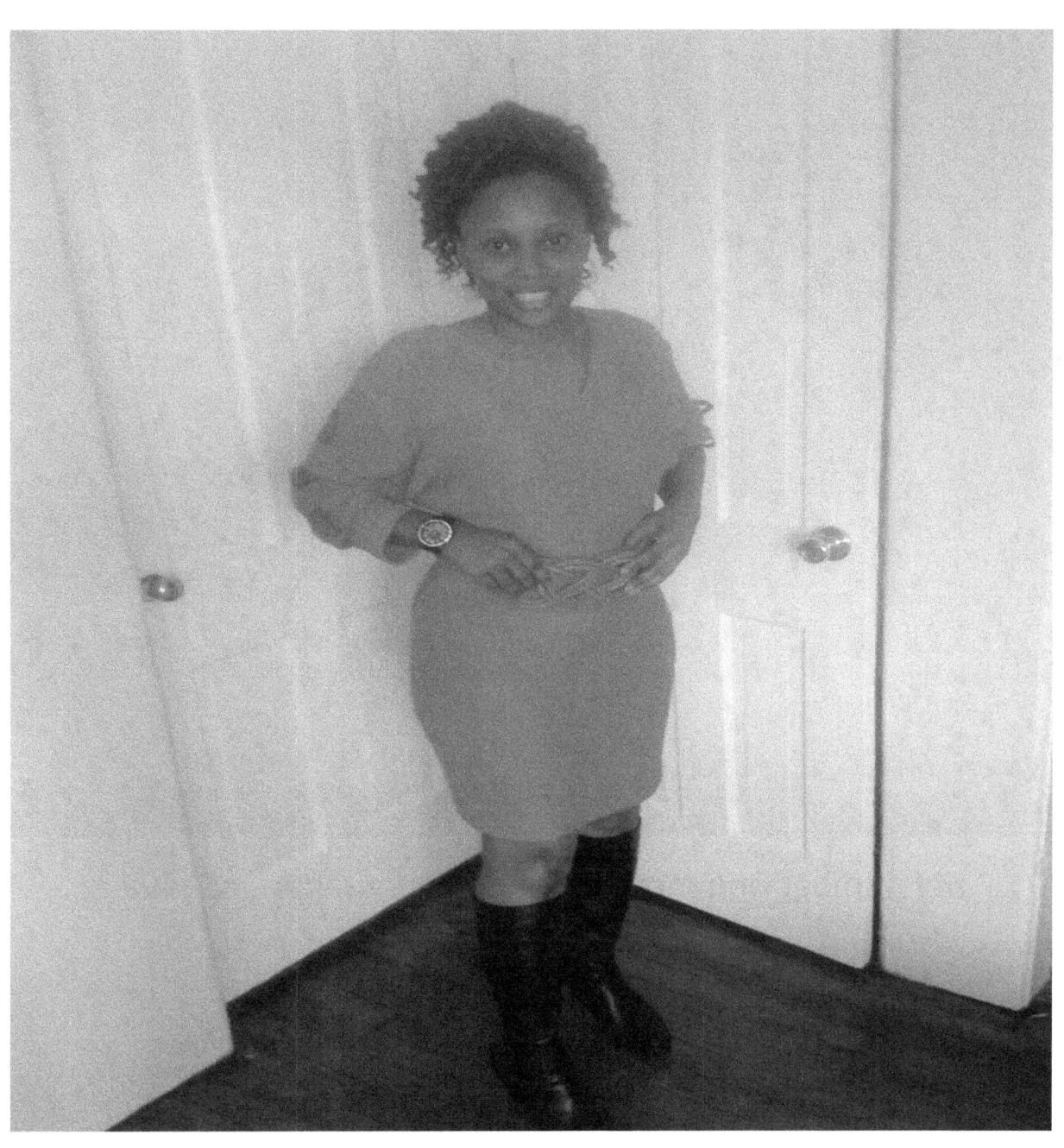

Feeling and looking good

Pretty in pink at my man's tree house ha

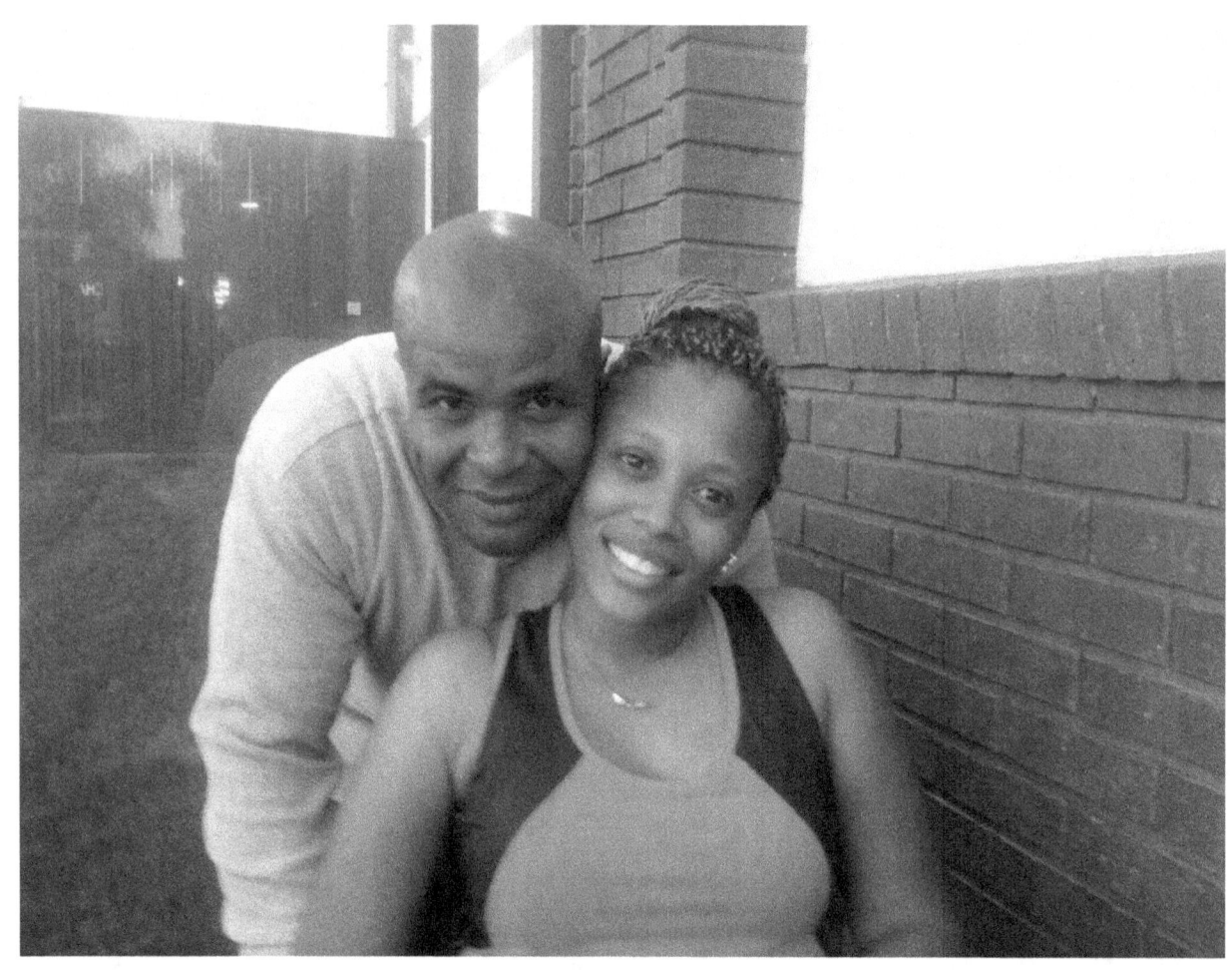

My number one motivator and encourager and love...

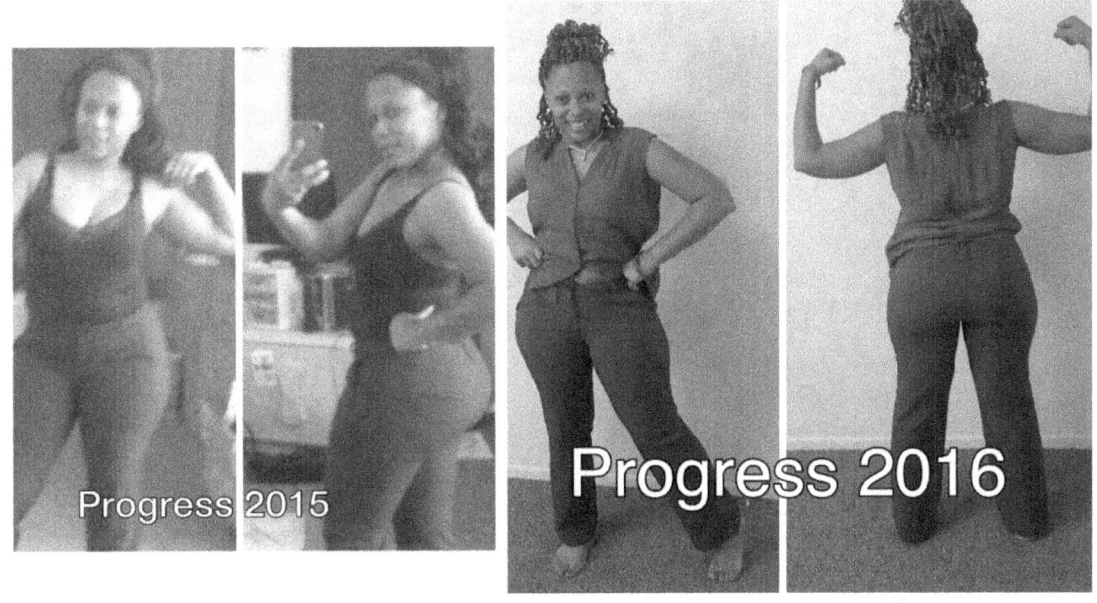

# It takes time to see results

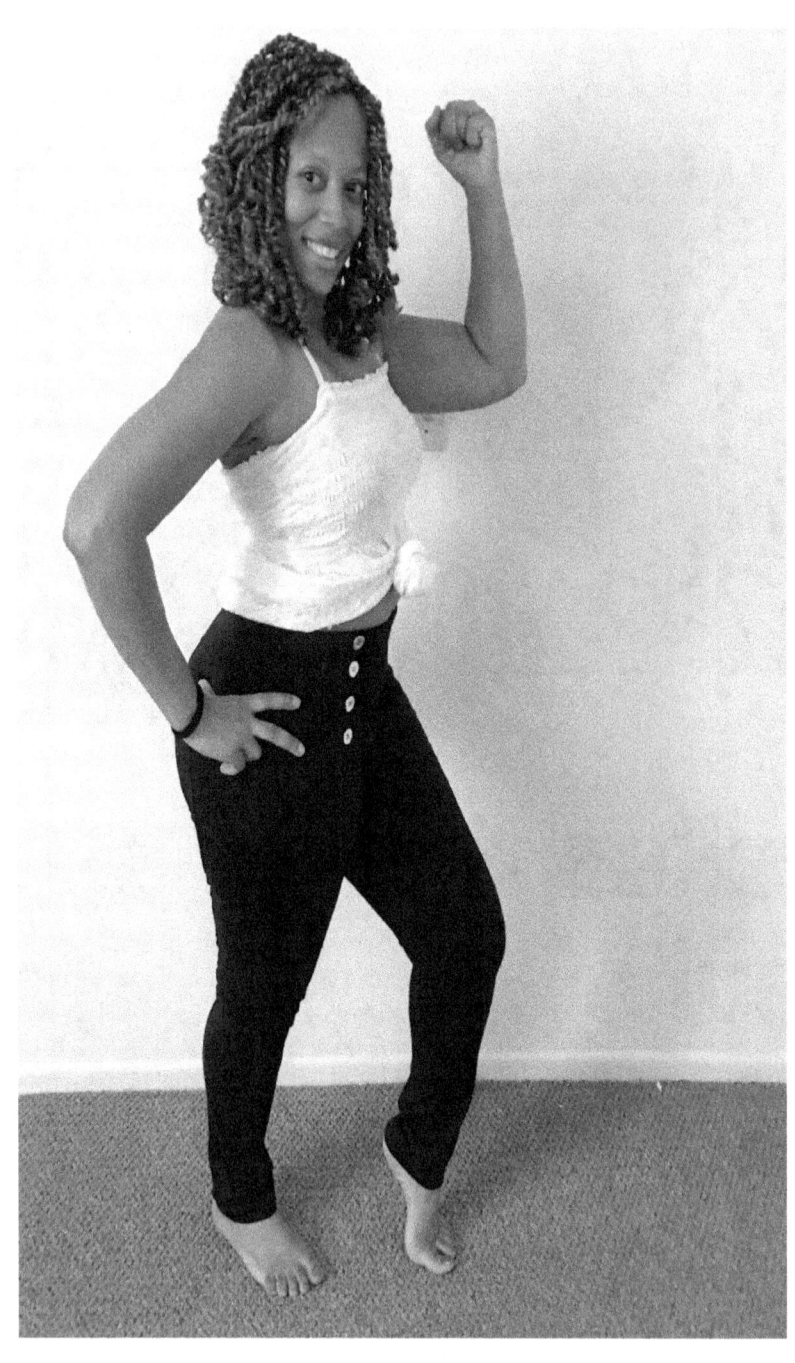

March 2016

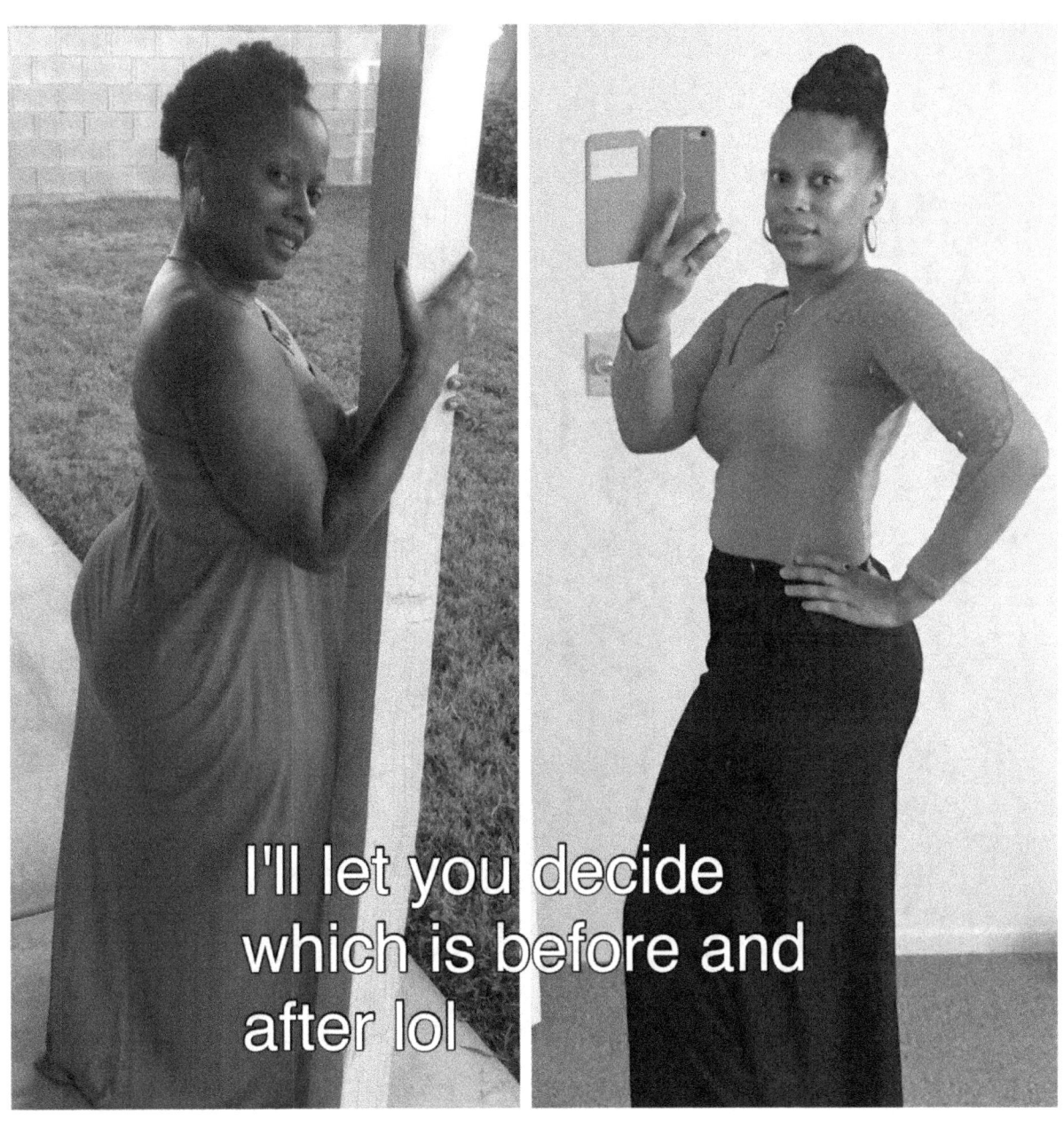

2015                                          2016

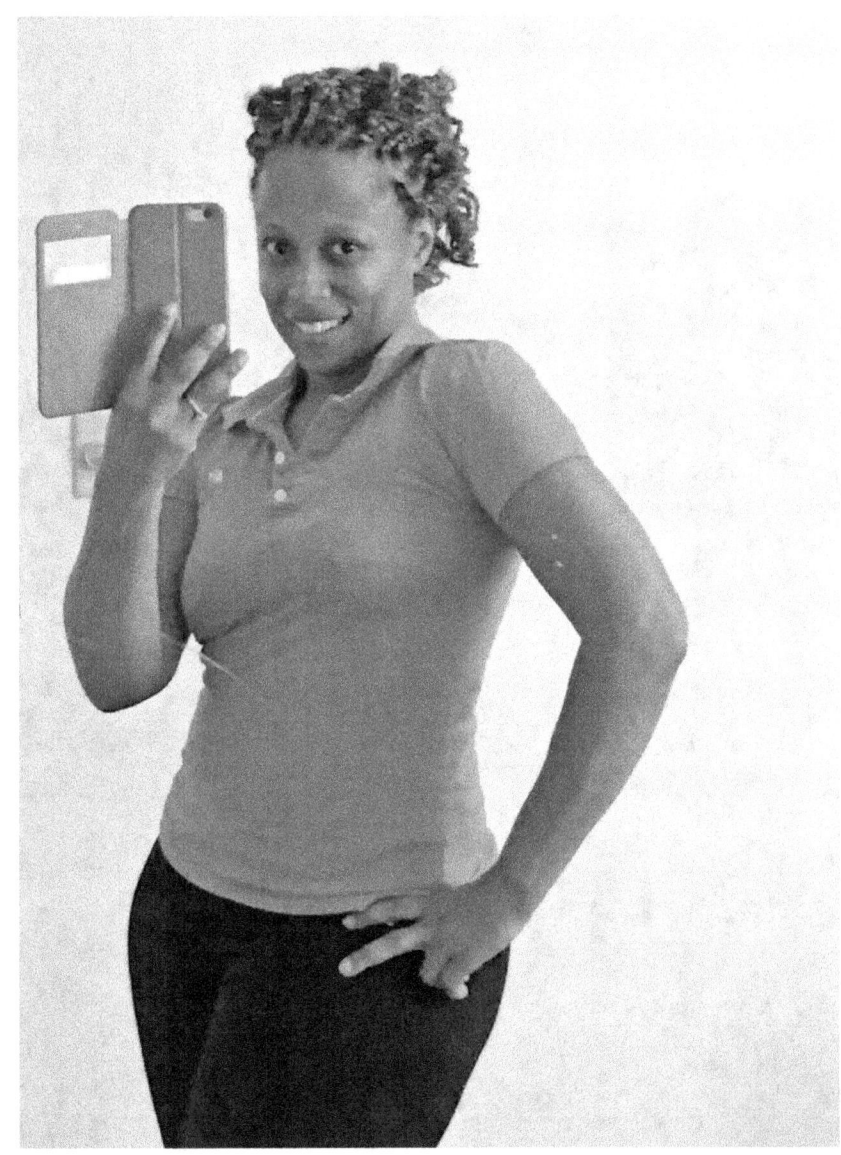

Had not worn that shirt in almost 3 years...

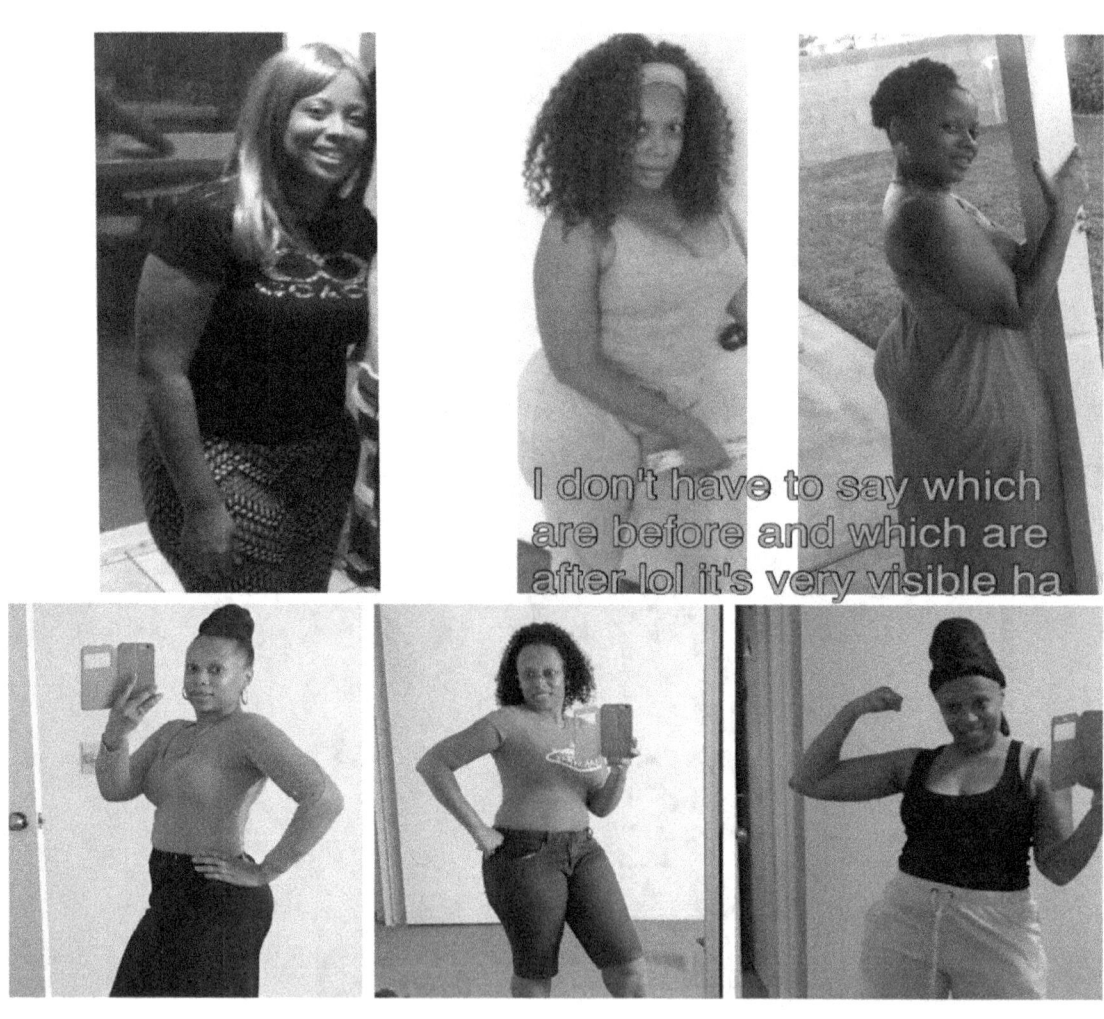

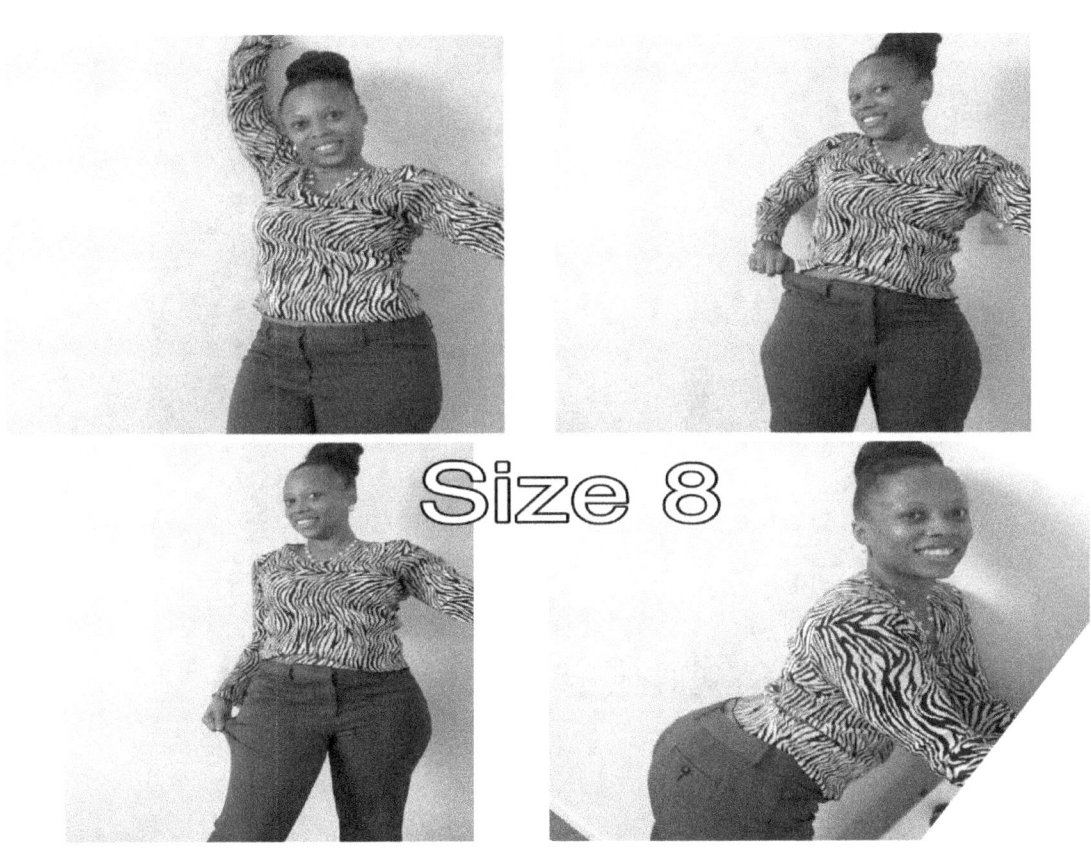

It has been almost 3 years since I wore an 8.

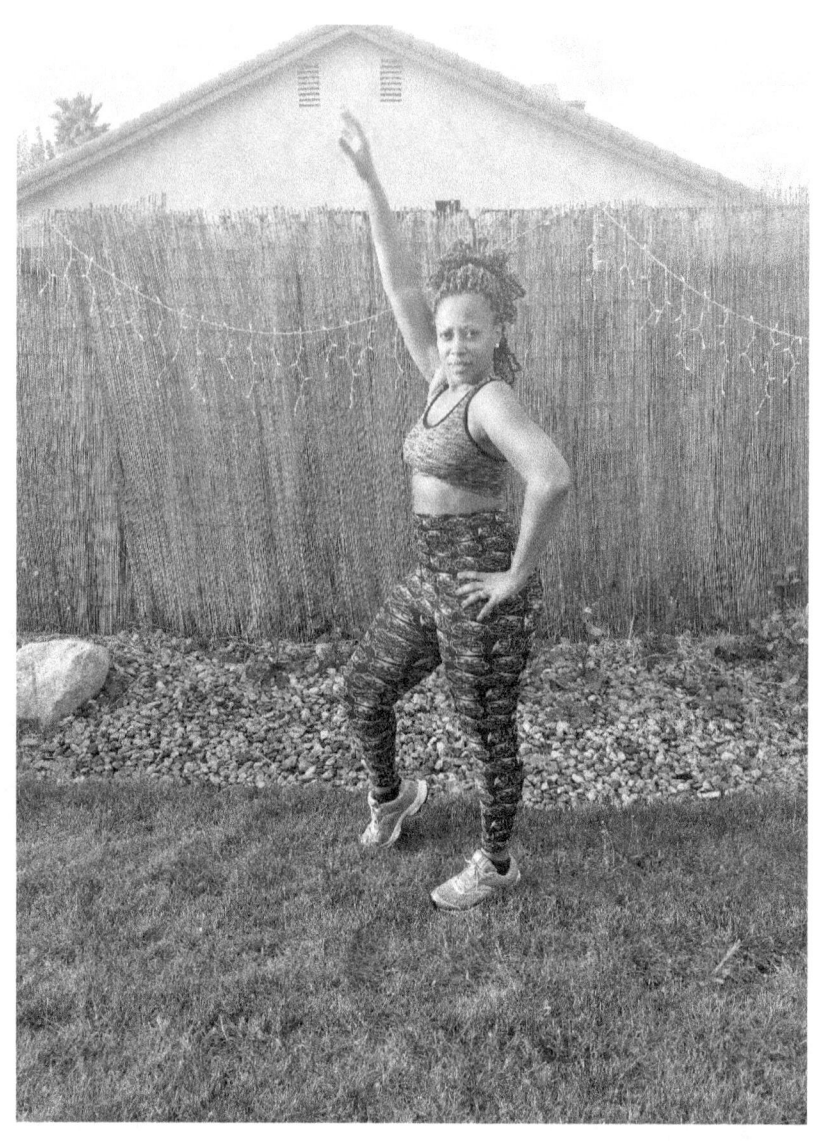

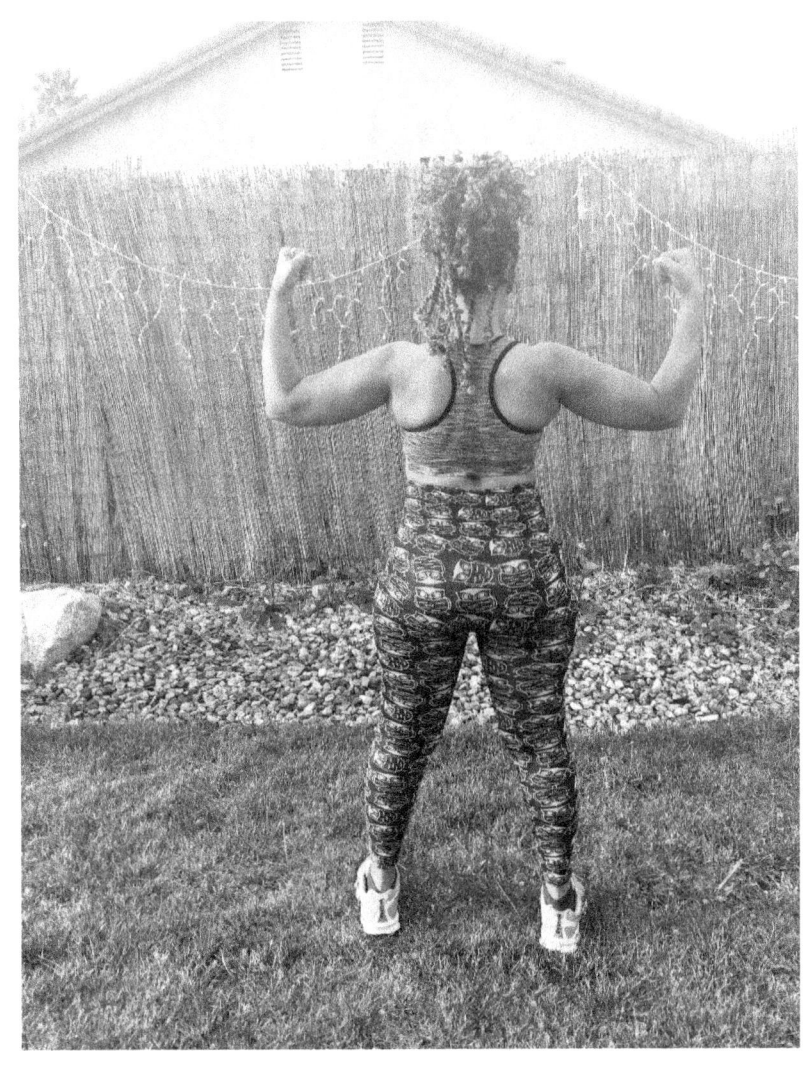

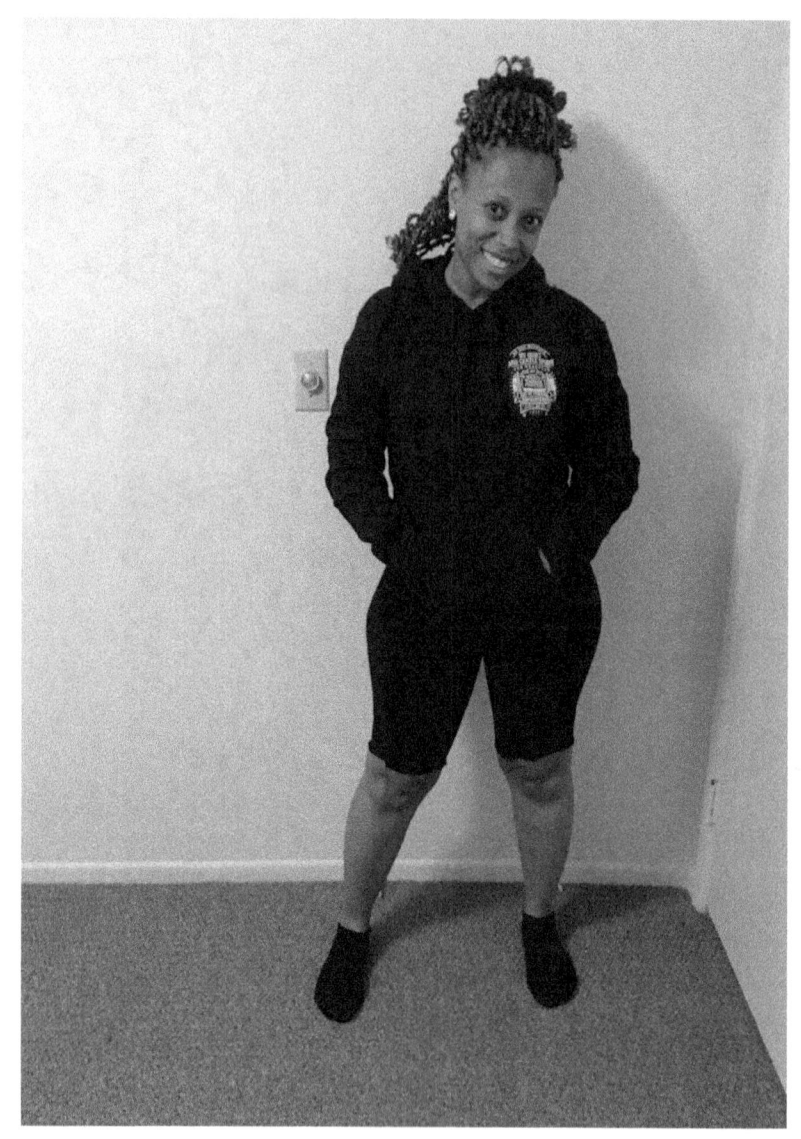

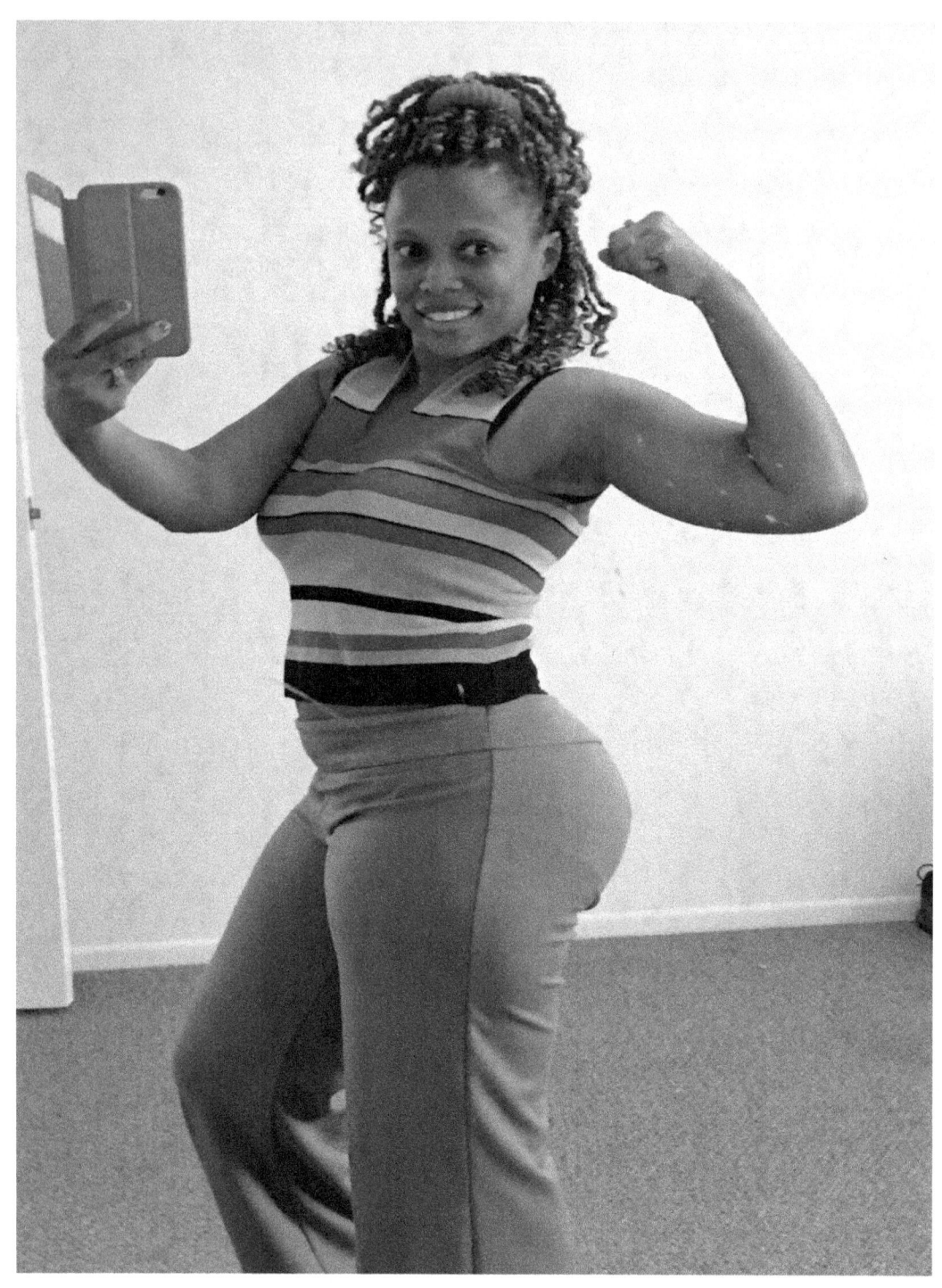

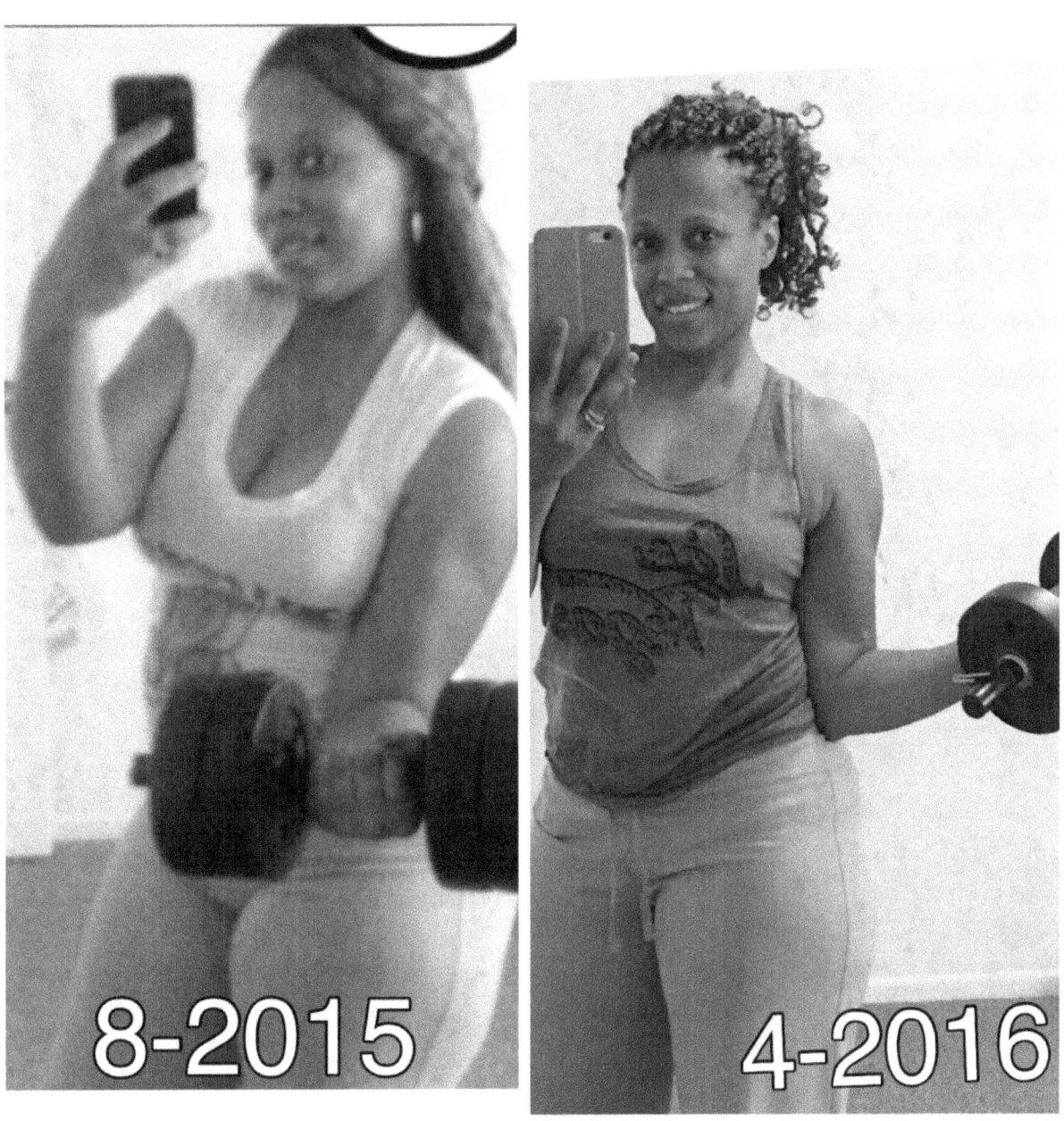

See, when you work out for different reason, your body does different things.

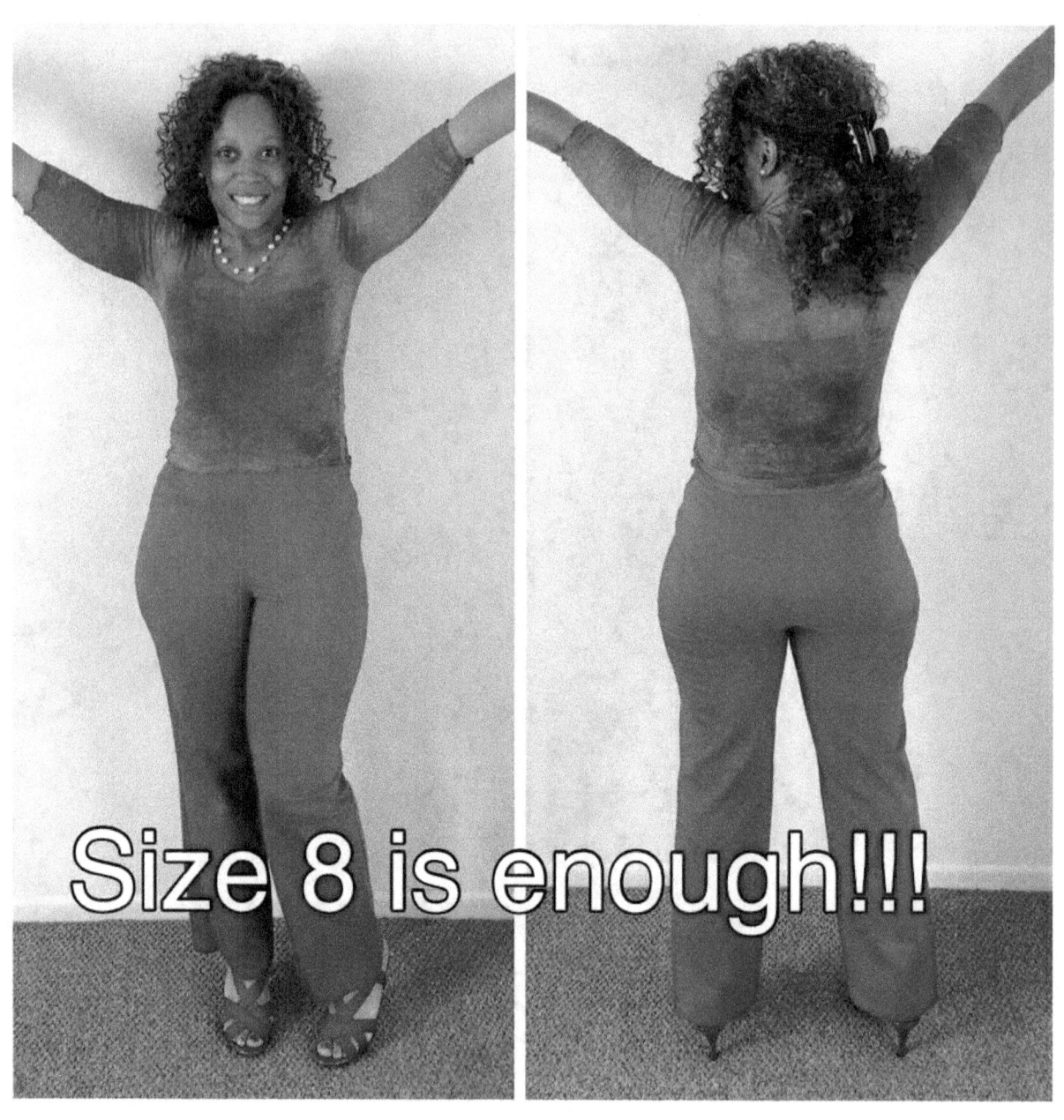

Size 8 is enough!!!

May of 2016—feeling great and loving life-- I had never been this size, I went from 4 to 16 so to now be 42 and a size 8 is GREAT!!!

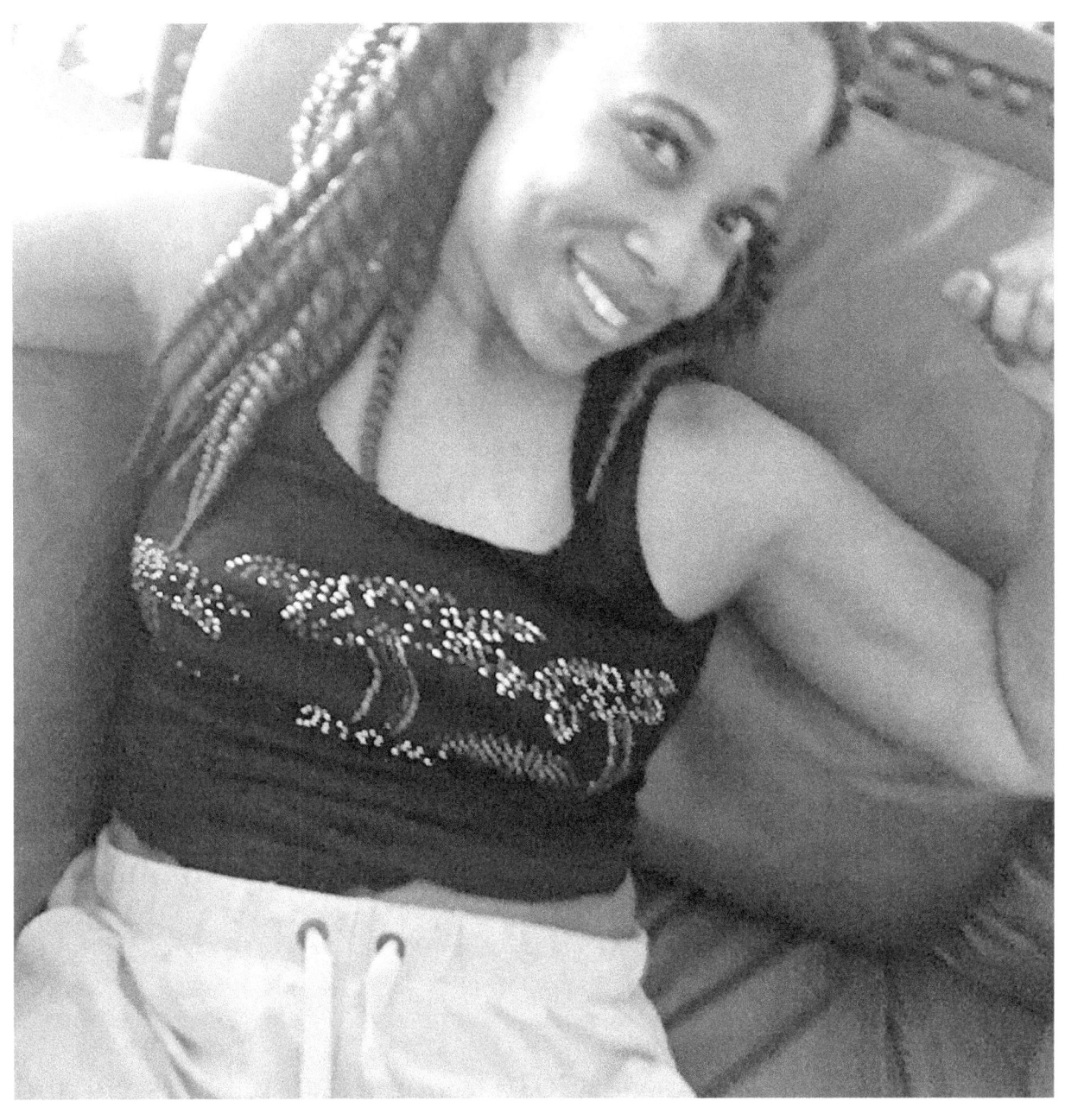

May 2016- the most recent version of me and I am loving it!!!

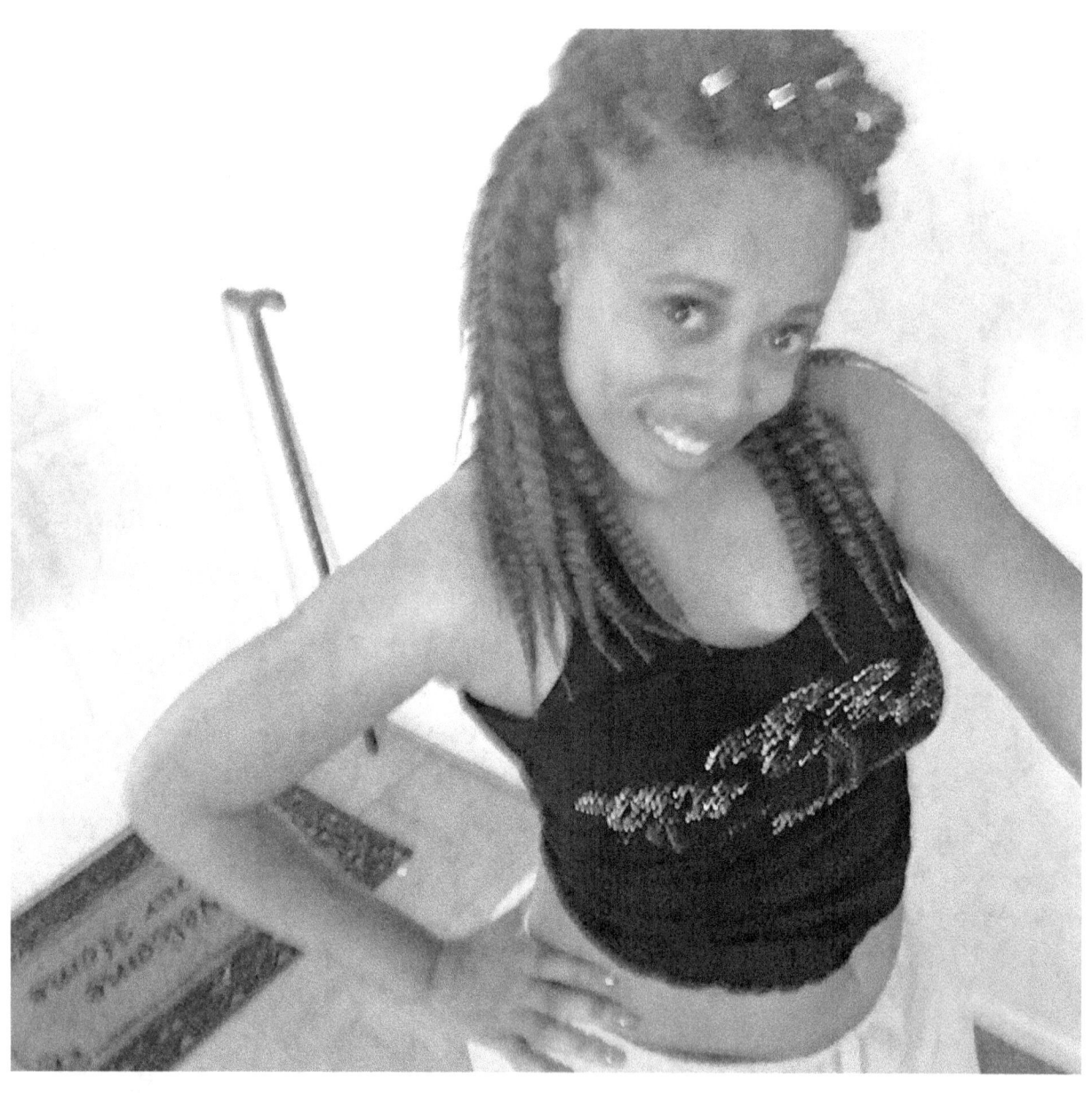

WHOSE THAT GIRL? HA, May 2016 loving the new hair style and body....

## Mind over body

Take it from me, there is nothing better than perfecting yourself. If you are not happy where you are, you can change.

It is up to you. No one else can make the decision for you but you. You make it up in your mind and you let your body know who is boss and make it happen.

I think back and think, what if I never decided to change, I would have missed out on so many opportunities and happy days.

Do what will make you happy and makes you excited about being you. You only have one life to live, so live it at your best.

If you are not sure how or need more help and tips just contact me on my public author page on face book or follow me on twitter and Instagram

More book info:

www.amazon.com/author/lockmarie

I also have more tips on my success story posted at

www.Shapefit.com/lockmarie

 a great website for inspiration and motivation from others who made it happen.

## Support and accountability

We all need someone to help us.

We all need someone to lean on.

We all need someone to be there to encourage us and push us forward.

Never feel you must do it alone.

Never feel you can do it all alone.

It does not have to be a family member.

It does not have to be a close friend.

Just a positive influence, is all you need.

Whether they are far or near, if you can daily get a text, note, call, email or kind word to let you know that you can do it and they believe in you.

I hate to say it, but it was not family that pushed me forward, it was strangers, friends outside of my regular circle that I was familiar with.

It was not the close friends but the associates and casual friends that I met that helped me stay on track and pushed me.

So sometimes it will not come from where you think it will, so do not get discouraged or upset. Do not stop and let that be a hindrance or distraction. Keep moving forward toward your goal.

# The
# End

www.ingramcontent.com/pod-product-compliance
Lightning Source LLC
Chambersburg PA
CBHW081224280526
45787CB00006B/2519